GW01465855

ONE MAN'S POISON

The 'Glucose' Factor

by

AMY MacGRATH

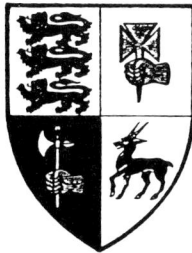

Published by Tower House Publications,
23 Primrose Hill, Tower, Co. Cork, Éire. Tel: 021-385720
1/22 Wolseley Road, Australia 2027. Tel: 02-3274052

ONE MAN'S POISON

© AMY MacGRATH

Published by Tower House Publications,
23 Primrose Hill, Tower, Co. Cork, Éire. Tel: 021-385720
1/22 Wolseley Road, Australia 2027. Tel: 02-3274052

Printed by Litho Press Limited, Midleton, Co. Cork, Éire.

1990

National Library of Australia Card Number and ISBN 0 9591879 2 8

All rights reserved. No part of this publication may be reproduced, stored in a retrieval system, or transmitted, in any form, or by any means, electronic, mechanical, photocopying, recording or otherwise, without the prior permission of the publishers.

This book is sold subject to the conditions that it shall not, by way of trade or otherwise, be lent, re-sold, hired out or otherwise, circulated without the publisher's prior consent in any form of binding or cover other than that in which it is published and without a similar condition including this condition being imposed on the subsequent purchaser.

Dedicated to industrial chemists and biochemists
all over the world, those I knew, and those who
were a voice on the phone, or a pen on the page.
Also to my very special family.

by

Amy MacGrath MA PhD OAM

Member of community bodies at various times -
school, university, hospital, theatre, club
Author of verse, plays, novels

The diagram below exemplifies the theme of the book

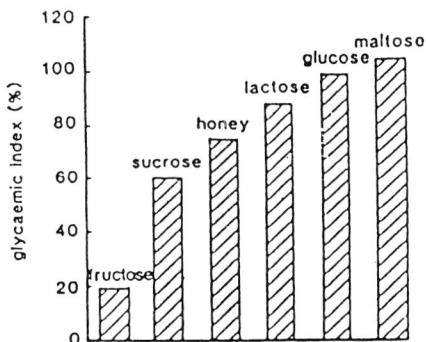

FIGURE 1.   THE GLYCAEMIC INDEX OF SUGARS

From 'Digestion and Absorption of Cereal Products- Fast or Slow'

J.C. Brand-Human Nutrition Unit, Dept Biochemistry & Public
Health

University of Sydney, N.S.W. 2006

Proceedings of a special symposium - Melbourne, Oct. 19 1987
with the 37th Annual Conference, Cereal Chemistry Division
Royal Australian Chemical Institute.

INDEX

TESTIMONIAL

by

Rosalind Atherton
Leone Lorrimer
Eloise McGrath Raw
Vivian Vivian

When confronted with a child screaming on the ground in front of an exasperated mother, we, the daughters of A m y MacGrath, would be likely to nod knowingly to each other, thinking as one *not* "It's the terrible twos", *not* "temper tantrums", but rather "He probably had Weetbix for breakfast!"

We survived the green birthday cake experiments of our childhood and have become, through the needs of our own children, earnest disciples of Mum's food discoveries. And we have all come to reflect in awe and gratitude for her long hours of patient enquiries and experimentation, for the years she spent baking bread for we four very hungry girls (and all our hungry friends!), and for the insults she bore at our expense for the sake of our health and wellbeing. In an era when mothers were (and often still are) treated as inadequate cretins and management of their children the source of all their childrens' ills, our mother's endeavours were a brave and enduring labour of love and patience.

Mum is a woman of enormous intelligence with unending patience and wonderful powers of observation developed through the rigorous training of three degrees in History. All of this applied to us as children led to answers which, in our humble but enthusiastic estimation, hold some of the keys for many paradoxical aspects of health and behaviour.

We, her daughters, have come not only to respect and treasure all her efforts on our behalf, but also to marvel at how well her discoveries work in application to our own children (all chips off our collective genetic block) and to ourselves again in our rediscovery of Mum's diet as adults.

We learned our dietary credo at her knee and have badgered her into helping us when our childhood problems surfaced in our own children. *We* were the exasperated mothers of screaming or chronically unwell children! In desperation we demanded answers for our children. In delight we discovered not only how well Mum's diet works with our kids but also how much better we are ourselves to return to the diet of our childhood.

We now run with renewed horror from Maltose/Glucose Syrup in all its manifestations (guaranteed to turn some angelic children into biting, thrashing, screaming monsters!) and never send the children (or ourselves) to school (or work) without a balanced breakfast! The effect on our children's temperament, concentration and health and, in turn, our own, has been nothing short of miraculous.

We commend to all parents - and especially the exasperated mothers of screaming children - our mother's wisdom.

FOREWORD

In March, 1968, my findings on diet were published in the Australian 'Journal of the Dietetic Association' (Victoria) after they had been brought to the attention of a conference of Australian Dietitians by Mrs. Venn Brown of the Bread Research Institute (C.S.I.R.O.). They were also mentioned in the Journal of the American Dietitians Association, Chicago, Vol. 51, No. 1.

The findings alleged maltose/glucose intolerance in my four daughters (then aged 6-14), enhanced by the prevalent use of 'glucose syrup' in processed foods, and sensitivity to grains unless fermented with yeast. These findings were the result of six years of 'blind trials', as foods were not labelled at that time.

The official notice of the Dietitians Association was immensely gratifying to me, as it lifted my persistent trials out of the category of food faddist. Not that anyone but myself cared. To everyone else but that growing band of industrial chemists, dietitians, and a handful of medicos, who had given vital pieces to the jigsaw, I was still just one of those diet freaks who were a symptom of the back-to-the-harmonies-of-nature movements of the exuberant sixties.

The deluge of new diets of this new wave, which has grown into 'health' food shops the length and breadth of the land, had already begun. The Adele Davis diet, the Pritikin diet, the Jarvis diet, and a host of others. The avalanche of books. Low fat. Low sugar. Whole grains. Low tannin. Low caffeine. Best sellers all of them.

And in their train the herbalists, the naturopaths. The do-it-yourself diets. The joke going the rounds of New York was close to the bone. Soon all a hostess would have to do was provide the dinner table, and everyone would bring their own special fad with them, the grape, the vegetarian, etc.

I was just one more apostle of some self-invented obsession. As the head of the paediatric section of the B.M.A. in the United Kingdom said when my local doctor put my theory to him, I was a paranoic obsessive, and a danger to my children who should be removed from my custody at the earliest possible opportunity. My local doctor had the wit to show me the letter. Time has, of course, shown otherwise.

In the meantime, the doctors could be forgiven for drawing their metaphoric skirts aside, while the public went on embracing this chaos of psuedo-scientific practice with an infinite proliferation of self-invented diets.

The biochemists simply went on with their patient, exacting, meticulous laboratory research- sometimes verifying, sometimes renouncing, former hypotheses, e.g. that high fat diet causes heart disease in the former case, or that sugar (sucrose) is bad, or that lack of sunlight is the prime cause of rickets in children.

In 1987 I was forced to do the same- to revive my research after a lapse of twenty years, as I now had four grandchildren aged 2-6, who more or less exhibited the same problems. One was worst of all with chronic asthma. My daughters, their mothers, demanded the answer I could not give.

Why was the low glucose, low gluten diet (except for white flour fermented with yeast) not 100% adequate in keeping allergy or personality problems at bay? The answer did not wholly lie in applying the diet with the most sensitive members of our genetic inheritance.

My daughters also demanded clearer layman explanations. They knew by their own experience that I had always been on the right track. They also knew I needed to be pushed forward along that track. Inconsistency remained in my working theory that required explanation. The inconsistency was as follows. Our sensitivity to wheat and its kindred grains was not absolute as with coeliac disease (an allergy to the gluten, or protein, of wheat).

For instance, we could eat wheat under certain conditions-
a) if wheat flour was fermented with yeast for six hours.
b) if such wheat flour was white, not brown or wholemeal.
c) if unfermented wheat starch was separated from its gluten protein, and then eaten alone, or recombined as cornflour with gluten.
I had no explanation for this paradox.

Yet I lived in a world governed by absolutes. Everyone around me made unqualified declarations such as 'I am allergic to wheat'. Such people would announce they were allergic to whole categories- dairy products, eggs, wheat, oranges, chocolates, cheese, and so on, without regard to the differential dynamics of such foods. There was no relativity.

8

You either could, or could not, tolerate whole classes of so called allergic foods, no matter how they were used in the diet.

A glorious ignorance reigned. No-one realised there was such a thing as dynamics in food. Mothers gaily brought up their children in an alarming state of food illiteracy. This would not have mattered a tinker's curse, if they had been following squarely in their ancestors' footsteps. Many were not. The new age of working mothers with a serious dependency on supermarkets had dawned. The quick food fix beckoned. Escape from kitchen drudgery. Escape from the dark age of their grandmothers' slavery. The result was improvised diets, unbalanced though they appeared to be, or sometimes balanced when they did not.

While mothers scanned the labels sedulously for the vices of 'additives', i.e. food that was not considered 'natural' as it had been chemically produced such as colourings, emulsifiers, etc. there were other threats that existed within the plants themselves that were never mentioned, and one at least that was not always correctly described, i.e. glucose syrup.

More and more of my friends and acquaintances had adopted the new holy writ- the more whole, the more wholesome; the more raw, the more nutritious. New fads swept through the community. Sesame seeds, Lebanese buckwheat, mung beans, germinating alfalfa. Oat bran. Pasta. Pizza. Restaurants bowed to these fashions. Airlines. It became impossible to get a white roll except on request, and that with difficulty. On the airlines, it could only be found in first class, which reminded me of the fact that only the wealthy in Ireland ate white bread. The Anglo-Saxon diet patterns of my forebears became unrecognisable.

All bowed to the new passions with only the sketchiest idea why they did so. They might thrive better by adopting these new fancies in place of the old tried and true diets of the past. Yet we had all clearly thrived on the diet they thought loathsome in the extreme- white bread, cakes, pastry, suet, treacle, less fruit and no nuts.

Was it the myth that man had moved from some harmony with his earth to the corruption of cities and civilisation? This was a myth fostered by those who spoke of ancient patriarchs living to great ages in remote valleys of the Caucasus or the Himalayas on simple diets; a myth of 'natural man' begun with the eighteenth century enlightenment casting its nostalgic yearning back to thoughts of a past communal golden age.

9

The cult of this 'sacred cow' among people of considerable acumen might have made more sense if they had spent as much time learning about their bodies over the years as they had spent debating the state of society, religion, or party politics.

But scarcely anyone could define the components of the food they so recklessly experimented with in the do-it-yourself diets let alone tell the difference between carbohydrate and starch, or either of these and protein.

The blissful state of ignorance among the intelligentsia is even more profound when it comes to the intricate transformation of food in the body from complex to simple molecules. I know because I was one of those I criticise, who simply knew nothing of this miracle of one's own life.

I was forced to learn in order to explain the riddle of my genetic peculiarities to my children. In doing so, I found myself putting my feet squarely back in the footsteps of my ancestors. The diet pattern my mother had followed (English and Irish) was far more suitable to my dietary problems than anything my health-conscious friends recommended. In contrast to theirs, we preferred old-fashioned white bakery bread, a wider range of non-wheat starches, an uninhibited use of butter and sugar, and well-cooked rather than raw food of any kind.

At this point no doubt health fanatics will cry horror, or dismiss me as a rare species. They will set this account aside without waiting to read my final conclusion that the old workhorses of the kitchen were right. They were the repositories of ancestral wisdom. They knew man is not naturally in harmony with his environment. They understood that most raw plant food is innately poisonous. They had the wisdom to neutralise that toxicity by skills developed over many centuries, skills we have wholly abandoned or, if we overcome them, do so by accident.

But this book is written first and foremost for my children, and for others to read as well if they will. It is meant to build them a bridge between the old and the new. However, I have found it quite impossible to explain why raw plant food can be toxic without first beginning with simple explanations and definitions of the most elementary facts so that they may revive ancient folklore in their diet.

How they may reconstruct it will be different, of course, from how a Greek or Turk may do so, because their derivation is Celtic-dominated. Celts were not basically wheat eaters until very

10

recent times- mid-nineteenth century- owing to the climate. Their intolerance of it as a dominating staple of diet (as it has become) is therefore much greater than that of anyone from the Middle East, where wheat has been cultivated for thousands of years.

Yet vastly dispersed populations- native, Asian, African- have food patterns and consumption habits that show they too had evolved ways to mitigate the hostile qualities of plants that were the predominant staples of their diets. It is also clear they lack as much adaptability as the Irish to modern diet, when the delicate balance of man to the poisonous potential of plants becomes overturned in the mistaken belief that the more natural the state, the more benevolent.

This book is about my journey back in time towards my British ancestors. This journey had three stages.

1. The years, 1972-7, when I developed a working family diet which alleviated the three major categories of symptoms - allergic, behavioural, neurological and hypoglycaemic.

2. The period, 1987-8, when I resolved the inconsistencies depending on how the plant was presented.

3. The pursuit of these facts in scientific journals to see if any light was shed.

No story of that journey is adequate for my 'laymen' children without insisting they must understand-

a) matter- whether of plants or humans- is not static, but a living pyramid of molecules, a multifarious miracle of atoms of carbon, hydrogen, oxygen and nitrogen.

b) the body is an incredibly involved factory engaged in converting food from complex to simple molecules, by which process tissue and bones are rebuilt, blood glucose from fuel manufactured, and glycogen banked up in the liver for blood glucose reserves.

They must know the language of this miracle, the names of its workforce, the stations of its highway.

I set this down for my children as simply as I can. If it is not simple enough, then I urge them to find a textbook which is, as they face rearing children in this food chaos of our times. Let me state categorically that I am at odds with most, if not all, textbooks, which consistently advocate foods in supermarkets, and health food shops, which I cannot buy.

I have concluded that man was originally more carnivore than herbivore. His system is more at ease with the proteins of animal flesh than with the proteins of plants which do not provide

11

the ten essential amino acids he requires in any one plant. This very inadequacy is a potent argument against asserting any dogma that man began as a plant gatherer, or for using that dogma as a philosophical basis for drastic change in diet from centuries of ancestral wisdom.

In an age when so many established concepts have been challenged, it is not surprising that established ideas about diet have not escaped. However, those who want to sweep aside all old modes of dealing with food should remember far more is at risk in abdicating from old food habits, than from old ideas. This stricture applies particularly to mothers, when they rear their young.

Far too many have abandoned their forebears' inexorable custom of having a good breakfast to start the day. Far too many have a hurried piece of toast, croissant, or plate of breakfast food, to break their long night's fast.

Far too many despise the solid sit-down family meal of my youth, when we invariably had cooked dishes- whether fish, eggs, or meat. We never went quite as far as the North Germans with their cheese and cold sausages to choose from as well, but we had the kidneys, the kippers and all the rest, and the porridge in winter.

But now I ask, whatever happened to breakfast? Mothers think it enough to shove a piece of toast in the hands of their children of tender years, or even not to shove it at all; to let them go to school with or without, breakfast as they fancy.

All too often working mothers leave them to get their own breakfast on a catch as catch can basis, as if children have the knowledge to give themselves a balanced diet. Rather they will do as they see their parents do.

I remember a survey in a primary school classroom a generation ago elicited the disturbing fact that more than half the children in the class started the day without a proper meal. Mothers have even been heard to boast they have trained their children to go without breakfast at all.

How do any of these mothers imagine their children can function properly without fuel to 'start the day well'? How do they imagine they will grow straight and true? What price are the working mothers, or the lazy mothers, exacting from the future generation? How indeed have they become so ignorant as to know so little?

Have they forgotten in their clamour for pay, jobs, equality, and rights, that their primary job is to rear their children properly? The answer is inescapable. They have renounced the kitchen, as a fate that enslaved their grandmothers, without a backward glance at the fact that there were virtues in that enslavement, not least continual good-health and the buoyant mind that goes hand in hand with that health.

THE CHILDREN

This book is not by a scientist, and does not pretend to be scientific, nor a universal prescription for anyone or anything. This book is an 'I am' book. It has to be, because it is simply the story of observation of myself, my children, and grandchildren over thirty four years- 1954-88. No more.

Why 1954? That was when my first child was born, the child I was told I would never have, the daughter that was the first of four daughters- 1954-62. Who am I then? A child of the Canberra public service, sixth of seven children, third of four daughters. My father was a public health doctor, head of his department, son of a Victorian commercial traveller, who, like many descendants of recent migrants, was leading the family out of trade and business into the mandarin class of professionals. My mother was a full-time mother, daughter of an ex-Quaker outback, then country, doctor.

I went to the University at barely sixteen. My father chose the curriculum. History not science, because I came second in the State in history, and nowhere in science. My science was deplorable, either by fault of my teachers or myself, or both. When I emerged at the end of first year University with a high distinction in geography, it did not seem to occur to anyone I might have talent in that direction. I ploughed on with history, which, with hindsight, was not such a disaster. History was still pursued by deductive reasoning, compared to the emphasis on inductive reasoning in science.

So what has all this got to do with problems that were to arise in my children? Everything. Original sin must be confessed from the first. In matters of biochemistry and nutrition I was a clean slate for the moving finger of fate to write on.

The finger of fate began to write in 1954, when I was delivered of a perfect baby daughter by a general practitioner. It was a natural childbirth without any flummery of blood tests, pre-natal classes or exercises. No ultrasound to cheer me with news of the normality of the foetus. No husband to cheer me on in labour. A mother, who appeared long enough to say 'Now you know', before she caught the P. and O. liner for London. This does not mean she was not a wonderful mother. She was. But my father had died suddenly a month before.

There I was, alone, with no relatives, a useless mother-in-law, the sketchiest knowledge of how to rear a child, and a library of three books. My Karitane handbook, written by Dr. Truby King, a friend of my father, who developed the Karitane 'science' of maternity in New Zealand. The ubiquitous Dr. Spock with his fatal contamination from psychology's morass of 'red herrings', which encouraged motherhood anarchy. A Health Department book on baby care routines based on the Tressilian method. No other advisers except the local clinic sister. No home care such as councils had developed in England. No wise friends. No knowledgeable sisters. Neither of my older sisters had children, and anyway were in the wilds of London and New Guinea.

I worked at first from the Karitane book, the only one to offer guidelines. It was soon clear there was no hit and miss about the stern rules of Karitane, particularly if mother's milk was scanty as mine was. The screaming baby must be weighed before she was fed, then after, to determine just how much was really coming from mother, as well as the bottle supplement. The total must be counted at the end of the day to compare with Karitane's oz per weight schedule. But on other matters- a baby overactive both ends- the books, that I thought were my road to salvation, were silent. Except to say let 'him' scream, or 'he' will get into bad habits; and love 'him', or 'he' will feel abandoned.

For the next five years, nothing went right. Karitane went into the rubbish bin. Spock followed. The Health Department book last, although it had some advice which was very up-to-date, as I remembered much later.

What went wrong? The child, Rosalind, grew, yes. But she was volatile in temperament, hard to settle to sleep, uneven in energy, restless, variable in bowel movements across the spectrum of mild abnormality, accident prone, given to a type of mild epileptiform seizure under certain conditions, and occasional visual dysfunction. She was often subject to infection, vomiting attacks, and tonsilitis, for which doctors far too often prescribed one of the new wonder drugs, some of which were later withdrawn from use.

Motherhood was not the peaceful, harmonious progression of my fond imagination. It was uproarious days and broken nights; nothing like the experience of smug mothers I knew whose babies would play happily with the same toy for hours, sit steadily in the one place for hours by day, or sleep steadily through the night. I retreated from patronising mothers, who made me feel I was simply unable to manage my child properly. I ceased to go out 'en

15

famille', or perhaps friends ceased to ask me out. Was I oversensitive? Back to the Bible of motherhood according to Dr. Spock. It was my fault. Never the baby's fault. What rot! How could a child have unpredictable bowel movements, and seizures with screaming, and tramping of the legs while lying down, from mismanagement of its emotions? What logical nonsense! I doubt if Dr. Spock ever sat at home day and night, single-handed on the motherhood job, experiencing the problems he so glibly solved or shelved by saying 'consult your doctor'. He was a driver who had never driven a car. The very thought got my Irish up. I wonder how he would have managed my problems with his 'firm, loving care'.

Why were these manuals so often written by a man, anyway? Was he the one left at home to thrust recalcitrant children into strollers, to battle with them in shops as their fidget fingers fiddled with everything in sight, or who struggled to 'get them down at night'?

My sympathies were with the mother in the same ward as myself when my second daughter, Leone, was born. She burst into tears when she heard her second child was also a boy, thinking her problems of management had to do with his sex. She said the only peace she had ever had with her firstborn was when she got into a motorcar and drove for hours. She thought it was a problem with boys. I assured her the problem of an overactive child was not confined to boys.

This time the redoubtable Dr. Simmons, who had attended me when Rosalind was born, had retired, but the routine of lying in was the same. A no frills birth attended by a general practitioner. However this child, a girl, was different in temperament- quieter, more settled, less likely to have collapses of energy or so-called tantrums. But she was similar in the tendency to experience infections, sudden rises in temperature, and eventually to suffer allergy, in her case a persistent bronchitis, particularly in winter.

By the time the older of the two, Rosalind, was four, I was still awaiting the predictable days and nights others boasted, the well-run nursery they appeared to have; and for the disorders already mentioned to disappear. Why, oh why, were these sudden shifts in mood and health; why these sudden outbursts of screaming, fuss, obstinacy, even violence, so unsympathetically dismissed in all the text books as 'temper tantrums', the 'terrible twos', the 'awful threes' etc.? Why this roller-coaster of energy, this fluctuation in vision or motor coordination, this disparate growth and pains in lower limbs, this twitching and itchy skin,

16

this bad colour and racing pulse, this tendency to have double vision and run into the sides of doors? Why were there so many soothing noises about stages of growing up, jealousy of younger children, and similar placebos to pacify anxious parents, to insult their intelligence? This parent was not pacified and was insulted.

This parent gradually said such talk was obfuscating piffle. This parent discarded every pyschological postulate and began to study the physical child, both of them. Why should I do so? Some obscure scientific gene? Some scepticism inbred by my parents from their chapel and Quaker background? Some rage certainly with all the pseudo-science that clung to motherhood like a parasite growth strangling a mother's true instincts, as child study moved into the laboratory. Perhaps the voice of my father dissuading me from psychology as an inexact science.

So what did I begin to see when I cheerfully threw away Dr. Spock, by now falling apart in every sense from its undeserved best-seller status, into the dustbin at the time daughter three, Eloise, was exhibiting the same symptoms?

First and foremost, that the alleged 'temper tantrums'
a) had a duration seldom lasting more than half an hour.
b) occurred with fatigue, fasting, and too crowded a program.
c) could pass to an involuntary stage when the child would lie down on the floor rhythmically kicking, screaming, and beyond verbal control.
d) were diminished by food, rest, or quiet handling, not by discipline.
e) were accompanied by physical symptoms- poor colour, dark circles under the eyes, changed pulse rate, disturbed eye movement or aspect- such as staring, rolling, or nystagmus.
f) presented with an idee fixe, that is a repetition of the same thought, demand, request or action. This symptom had a fairly short time limit.
g) left no memory of 'naughty' behaviour in the child afterwards.

The first person I met who supported the view that 'temper tantrums' had a physical cause was a Woolloomoloo clinic sister (Health Department). She suggested such episodes might be treated as convulsions with cool packs on the head. My own method had been warm baths, and a cool flannel on the forehead, more often than not combined with an immediate offering of food. I was only to learn much later that the last was the best, since the episodes were in fact hypoglycaemic. However for some strange reason the baths did help.

17

In other words, tantrums were not to be treated as a pyschological issue of doing battle with the child by punishment, reproof or verbal argument. Whatever 'naughtiness' appeared on the surface, whether screaming, crying, jibbing, or propping, should be regarded simply as a physical response of the child to a hostile environment until physical answers were exhausted, or could be explained in terms such as birth trauma, mental illness, or disease. It should never be treated as a matter of bad behaviour, and therefore of discipline.

What then was the problem? Why did it cut across separate categories- emotions, digestion, allergy- which were normally all approached as distinct specialties? What did nystagmus of the eyes have to do with steatorrheoa or bronchitis? Questions that had as yet no answers, that led to a dead end until one day Rosalind, then five years old, said she had cramps in the stomach, a symptom long too familiar to myself.

Despite my general disillusion with the medical profession at this stage- through no fault of its own that I could see- I mentioned this to my local practitioner at King's Cross, Dr. Grieve, the doler-out of anti-biotics, who suddenly said the cramp in Rosalind's stomach could be allergy, and to watch what she was eating. How he came to open the locked door of my ignorance I will never know. Perhaps he had just been reading some account in his medical journal when I happened along. But then and there he handed out the first key. He had suggested a positive way to search for an answer, instead of merely recording negatives. It was somewhere to begin, a beginning I would never have made alone because I would never have thought to associate stomach cramps with allergy.

So what were the chief allergies in vogue at the time? What was the state of the art? Primitive, it seemed. Skin tests on the arm, which sometimes worked, so the mothers said, but not for us. Or withdrawal of foods by trial and error? Trial full of error as we soon found, since any trial depended on a busy mother's observations of response to the popular allergic fancies of the day- milk and its products, egg whites, pineapple, tomato, house dust, and pollen. At this stage I did not even know such causes of allergy were called allergens, or that they were held to be 'foreign proteins' that found their way into the blood to cause an immune response. But at least the allergists had a physical approach to medical problems. They were not concerned with psychological hypotheses.

My first reaction was that this way lies madness. However, with time and patience, a pattern of reactions with a logic to them became clearer. They would occur at certain times after meals, at distinct times of the day, on isolated occasions such as after birthday parties, or after particular foods. Some specially strong reactions stayed in mind. However mostly no reaction was as flagrant as asthma. Despite these decided observations, there was still no common thread, no apparent correlation between items in the range of food incriminated- as between Ovaltine, ice-cream, wheatmeal biscuits, salines, Paladac child tonic, cordials and so forth.

Rosalind was nearly eight, and Leone six at this time. They had grown normally, were above average in intelligence, and had survived most childhood ailments like chicken pox and measles unscathed. But they were still unsettled sleepers, prone to hives, skin problems, infections, poor colour and so on. But I also had two younger daughters as well by now- Eloise aged two, and a newborn, Vivian. These girls were already presenting with all the same initial problems, while the youngest was even more sensitive to milk, and had to be weaned onto a soya milk formula by the time she was one year old due to a continual loss of weight, and affectation of adenoids so serious they had to be removed.

Number three had 'temper tantrums', 'idee fixe' episodes, logical disorientation at times, changes in energy, appearance and colour, digestive disturbance, all even more pronounced than her oldest sister at the same age. She could stop in her tracks like a mule. Walk off and leave her, the wise ones said. You try it, I thought in my despair, and see if it works. Of course not. She had to be carried or pushed in a stroller until her fatigue balance was restored, and her mood passed off.

I learnt that diabetics could behave in this manner if they gave themselves an overdose of insulin, thereby precipitating hypoglycaemia. For example, my gynaecologist knew of a diabetic colleague, who drove through a red light after overdosing, then abused the police who arrested her. Similarly a diabetic in Hobart broke into a prohibited area with a dangerous disused radio broadcast tower and began to climb it. I could see I must be thankful for small mercies. All Eloise did was demand such things as butterfly wings made with string before she would go to a birthday party next door, or insist on the one and only forever same seat in the car. And her episodes were self-limiting.This stage in my life, preoccupied as I was with four children, I remember as a blur of

19

constant apprehension as to what might happen next. It would have been impossible to combine any valid career with mothercare. Such an option would have been grossly unfair to the children.

There was a distinct advantage in not being a working mother. My mind was not distracted by courses of study, part-time jobs, or responsibilities at work. I had time to sit and chat with other mothers, a vital part of maternal education that most working mothers miss out on. Due to this fact I invited another mother home to lunch one day. I did not know her particularly well as she was a working mother, a cellist teacher at the Conservatorium. I offered her sandwiches. She refused. She was a coeliac, she explained. She was allergic to wheat. To wheat? The bread of the Bible? The staff of life? The universal food, the one food I had never questioned?

Wheat? My mind began to spin backwards. Could I, or my children, possibly be coeliacs? No, every expert said. A coeliac is thin, spindly in build, with a blown-up stomach, and suffers from constant diarrhoea due to the damage to the layer of cells lining the small intestine. It was common for a coeliac baby to die from malabsorption until a scientist named Dicke discovered in 1952 that the protein, gluten, present in wheat, oats, barley and rye, was toxic to those suffering from this disorder. A coeliac, it seemed, was prone to infection, allergy, irritability and mental effects if wheat or its allied gluten grains was ingested- as we were. And yet we did not present with the serious life-threatening profile described. Could there be such a condition as mild coeliac disease, which did not exhibit the whole force of its lethal profile?

Now my head was eternally a refuse bin of facts- stories of many discoveries due to observation rather than formal experiment, as of smallpox, cholera, anthrax, the vector of the mosquito. What was so different about starting an empirical study, first with myself and then with the children, to see if gluten allergy was our problem? Would we not do as well as a cageful of rats? Or better? Such a study could only be an extension of what I had done with increasing futility over the years- withdrawing foods for a time, and observing the difference brought about by withdrawal. But these trials had been with foods used episodically, not with a food so ubiquitous in western diet as wheat, the main source of gluten.

Could my failure have been because the allergy did come from an all-pervasive source like wheat, more all-pervasive than it had been even in my childhood with its winter porridge, other-

20

starch puddings, etc.? If so, why were my symptoms more violent in my twenties than in my childhood? This qualification, doubt if you like, lingered in my mind as I faced the experiment of excluding wheat from our diet. The year was 1962.

THE PROBLEM

I rang the dietitian at Royal Prince Alfred Hospital, Miss Rogers, to ask for details of the coeliac diet. Much to my surprise, she did not ask for a doctor's referral, but took me on trust. She sent me a copy. I was appalled. I must exclude not only wheat, but also oats, rye, barley and millet; and must substitute wheat or maize cornflour (together with soya flour) for all wheat flour in bread, cakes and pastry. Cornflour? Dead white flour that I had been taught to scorn? Where was the food value? In soya flour it was true that there was some, but there was little soya flour in the recipes. I was so horrified that, even if I had been tempted, I would never have had the courage to try it on the children. I had so often read that white flour had little nutritional value, stripped as the experts said it was of nearly all its vitamin and mineral content.

There was only one answer. Try the coeliac method of cooking on myself, and see if it provided the magic key to the many symptoms of my twilight world between good and bad health. So I began, all unaware of the quite extraordinary path I was about to follow. Within a week the change was melodramatic.

Two things were obvious first. I did not feel tired by eight o'clock in the evening, nor in bursts during the day. I no longer had that perpetual feeling of never being quite well, of living with brakes eternally on, of enduring for want of knowing how much better I could feel. I felt like rushing out to announce this dramatic change to the world. I was Archimedes in his bath, Newton with his apple.

Other improvements followed. No more masked vision, as if peering through a very thinly opaque liquid. No more swollen eyelids, or red eyes. No more colonic spasms, and other unwanted digestive variations. No more occasional vomiting attacks. No more itchy skin. No more sinusitis from dust, perfume, pollen, etc. No more bouts of drastic hayfever to humiliate with endless sniffling nose, sneezing, spells of total incapacitation in bed. No more sweating or labile temperatures. No more continual roadblocks in concentration, lapses in sequential thinking. It was a miracle, a healing.

The scale of this healing could only have one possible meaning- that wheat did not merely affect the lining of the intestine but also the entire metabolism. The implication of such a conclusion was mind-blowing. If our problem was not coeliac disease, as people said, why did we respond to coeliac diet? Was there some other as yet unidentified factor in wheat that accounted for that other class of people affected by wheat, vaguely described as wheat allergics? People who walked round, as I had done for so long, half-bombed out with inhalants or anti-histamines?

Much later a medical friend, a research scientist, said I was asking these questions a generation too early. Twenty years too early in fact as it eventually proved. He was absolutely right. The biochemist's world of brilliant research was not moving forward quite so fast in the post-war world as I would wish.

One thing was soon clear- though I would shout to the world, the world would not hear. I was on my own, and would have to stand by my findings alone. Doctors were rightly cautious of unknown, untried propositions. They were two a penny. Doctors were rightly wary of laymen with propositions, even if arguable, since their profession was under siege from alternative medicine with its lunatic fringe against chemicals, additives, and pollutants. Moreover, partly in self-defence, partly from custom, the practice of medicine had become heavily weighted to findings made in the laboratory or field by 'specialised' professionals using selected samples carefully defined and studied under controlled and comparative conditions with either people or animals. This practice had accelerated with the advent of anti-biotics, but also sprang from the whole apparatus of standards of promotion and quality of research.

It became crystal clear that, as noone knew anything about the subject, I would have to start from scratch, looking at the facts and seeing what deductions could be made if necessary. The method of historians in fact, a method to which I had some pretensions with two degrees in history (a third came later). What was scratch? In this case, switching all four children off wheat, and eventually such small quantities of oatmeal, barley and rye as they ate, because presumably the same factor, whether or not it was in the carbohydrate or the gluten, would be in all these comparable grains.

To eliminate these gluten grains from the diet, believe me, was easier said than done. If you do not believe me, try yourself. Switch off all your entrenched food habits learnt long ago at your mother's table, leaving out the breakfast toast, the sandwich, pizza, pie or quiche for lunch, the cakes for afternoon tea, the bread rolls for dinner. And then imagine explaining to children aged variously eight, six and two, that they must refuse the food all other children around them were eating. Think how worried you, as a parent, would be at the effect of making the children feel 'different', of putting them on a diet without support from any doctor, or any known popular principle, and without any answer to friends who asked 'why can't they eat wheat?' We could hardly say they may, or may not be, coeliacs.

The diet demanded a new ethos, measuring everything with a diabetic scale, adopting the old style of mixing as my mother knew it- making up baking powder but substituting glucona-delta-lactone for cream of tartar as a raising agent with the bicarbonate of soda. There were saving graces. David Jones at that time sold a 'coeliac' bread, and health food shops- now tentatively springing up- sold 'gluten-free' bread, cake and pastry mixes, made by Barton Addison. Never mind that the bread crumbled at the touch of a knife, and had to be glued together literally by the butter, or that the breadmix, more plaster of paris than food, looked unutterably unhealthy.

There was another saving grace. My older children were remarkably co-operative for their years, perhaps because I harped on the theme they were involved in an experiment which could be enormously important for the future of other children (a tale I did not believe then for a moment); perhaps because they were highly intelligent, and understood they not only felt better, but they also immediately lost their various minor complaints- Leone her persistent cough and raw skin around the finger nails; Rosalind her hives, nystagmus etc. Most important of all they lost their fluctuations of energy as I had. Their metabolism evened out, as if they had had what I called a 'pre-diabetic' condition with unstable insulin levels and lost it. I no longer had to carry a stroller around as insurance against collapse of energy, as I was still doing for the younger ones.

I had always feared diabetes. My grandmother died in a diabetic coma in her fifties in 1921, my grandfather of diabetes mellitus. And it was possible this propensity lurked in my husband's family history also. I suspect so, in view of the fact all my children seemed to have inherited the puzzling problem.

During the first year, I still had no solution for the fact the diet was an unqualified success, despite the evidence that my children were demonstrably not coeliacs with the bloated stomach, excessive diarrhoea, occluded intestinal villae, spindly arms and legs, which were the clinical medical picture. Their stomachs were flat. Their digestion veered at times towards constipation

24

(fluctuating either side of normal). Their growth was average. Why therefore should they respond so dramatically to the coeliac 'gluten-free' diet? Was there such a thing as a minor coeliac condition? Was this a new correlated condition? Or did the coeliac condition have another aspect to it as yet unidentified? I set out to find the answer.

Doubting myself, I paid good money to see a paediatrician. He was dismissive and insulting saying 'your children are not coeliacs', although I had already said that myself, merely adding the one qualification, that they responded to the diet for some unknown reason. He was the kind of male doctor feminists love to hate. Some time later, my much more open-minded British trained general practitioner from King's Cross had an even worse reaction when he sent my notes to a friend, the then head of the paediatric section of the British Medical Association in England, who wrote back to say I was a paranoic obsessive, and my children should be taken away from me at the earliest possible age. Diagnosis by correspondence! I still have the letter. My children remain a close family I am thankful to say, and now besiege me with demands for definition and detail, as their children have inherited the condition.

There was no doubt from the first of the efficacy of the empirical approach. Apart from the immediate appearance of good health in the children, there was other evidence. The headmistress of Sydney Church of England Girls Grammar School commented how much my oldest girl had changed, saying 'she used to be such a bad-tempered girl'. This observation seems remarkable, as she was only eight, and the school had nine hundred pupils, although there was another reason for taking notice of her. Both she and her sister were performing so well, she advised me to change them to Woollahra Opportunity School where they would have more competition than in the much smaller junior school where they were.

My second daughter improved in other ways. She lost her lethargy, absent-mindedness, and other auxiliary troubles like nasal discharge and gumboils.

The months wore on. I acquired some expertise in minute shifts in the childrens' mood and appearance. So it was that I noticed a change in Rosalind every Sunday after her regular outing with Alderman Ayres and his family. For weeks I questioned her as to what she had eaten. The answer would be ice-creams, milk-shakes, drinks- nothing which was on the coeliac prohibited list we had followed to date. Puzzling! These items did not contain the gluten, which was anathema to coeliacs, nor did the sweets in grandmother's perpetual lolly jar, which seemed to affect my two year old after every visit. So what could possibly be offensive about them? The amounts seemed to be harmless. The grandparents were restrained, well aware of the flood of propaganda about dental caries from sugar, which led to fluoride campaigns. I did not think the children had an intolerance to sugar per se. Their excellent response to 'coeliac' cookery, based on sugar, would argue against incriminating sugar. I dabbled with thoughts of fructose. But the same still applied.

The answer did not seem to lie with additives, the current 'villains' in food for which Dr. Feingold was responsible. My children were not the hyperactives he had in mind. He had a point, of course. In the drift from home cooking to a supermarket based diet with a switch to an 'instant' kitchen, I, like so many other mothers, was offering my family a great many prepared foods and drinks that were never available in my mother's day. There were some things among them to which my children reacted more than others- artificial green drinks, salines, coloured 'cheesels', and bright 'pink fairy floss'. But doubt hovered over other foods that could not be satisfactorily explained by the parameters of the 'additive' lobby.

Now at this point, I happened to notice that my third daughter was affected by the Minties that Grandma had in continual supply in her quarters- not remarkably so, but markedly so. I tracked the Minties down to Sweetacres. The telephonist put me onto Mr. Jarman in the laboratory. His first response merely gave me the answer I knew already. There was no gluten in Minties. But when, still troubled, I rang again, I must have asked him if there was anything else that could give trouble, because he gave me a different reply. Did I know what went into sweets? I said sugar, of course. Bear in mind there was no labelling of sweets then. He said not quite. Sweets also contain glucose syrup.

I was astounded, and asked what on earth glucose syrup could be, imagining of course that he meant the glucose then known as dextrose. He said not exactly. Glucose syrup was a general description for a whole range of syrups of different 'conversions' produced by chemical engineering, wherein glucose (dextrose) was to be found with malto-dextrins in variable proportions according to the end result desired. Clearly the designation glucose syrup was highly misleading to a layman like myself fondly imagining the

26

glucose being offered was dextrose in a syrup form; and must deceive many who read it so often on so many labels in supermarkets today.

I asked Mr. Jarman why glucose syrup was used in sweet manufacture. For various reasons, it seemed. For cost, viscosity, shelf life without spots or stickiness. Even as he spoke, I remembered all those sticky sweets of my childhood being doled out from big glass jars into white oiled paper bags, and how you had to lick your fingers after you ate them. Sweets made of sugar, like home-made sweets. I could not recall having had any reactions from these sweets, but then our bags of sweets were so much smaller in those days. Could the fact my children had some reactions be due to the fact the children were eating glucose syrup, or bigger bags of sweets, or both?

Mr. Jarman offered to bring me a sample of glucose syrup to try out with the children. I asked 'why would you go to this trouble for me?' He said 'I like a challenge!' But perhaps the curiosity of the true scientist was awakened. He was as good as his word, and brought me a jar of the syrup, which I was surprised to find was a fairly tasteless viscous substance. I gave Rosalind a flat dessertspoonful. Two things happened. She had temperament within the hour. She demanded more, indeed tussled with me to get the bottle. Needless to say I hid it, and asked more questions.

What was this glucose syrup? A product made from wheat starch by enzymic or acid engineering, after the gluten was extracted, and used either in dry powder form or viscous form in the food industry. A product considered so harmless that it was being widely incorporated into many supermarket foods; to such an extent that both Arnott's biscuits and Sweetacres only had three varieties each which did not contain it. But none of them were labelled to say so. Therefore any test I intended to make to see whether the children were being affected by glucose syrup would have to be entirely by blind trials. This was to take years.

THE VILLAIN

Because 'glucose syrup' had now entered the picture as a major factor in our debate as to why the gluten free diet worked or not, I was obliged to leave the safe launching pad of the coeliac diet with its prescribed parameters, and leap out into blank space as it were without any parachute. I spent the next two years working back over the whole inventory of food. It was surprising how often glucose syrup appeared as a common factor in many foodstuffs, such as medicines or icecream, that were not apparently related.

Was glucose syrup, this allegedly natural substance, a toxic factor in its own right? If so, was it a variable toxic factor according to the complementary intake of food? Was it a co-factor with gluten, or an entirely independent factor? These were questions that demanded painstaking answers.

The only possible method of finding such answers was to persist in the gluten-free diet, and to add or withdraw foods known to contain no gluten but which could potentially contain glucose syrup, and observe any difference in response. These would, of course, be blind trials, except in the case of sweets, as no foods were labelled, and I still had no real comprehension how widely glucose syrup was being used in foods where you would least expect it to be. The full horror of that revelation had yet to come.

At the point I began this research, my eldest daughter refused to eat the gluten free bread any longer, and for six weeks returned to eating ordinary white bread. She was then ten years old. She plunged from top of the class in almost every subject to middle of the class. The intellectual drop was so conspicuous, that the headmaster was prepared to give me a certificate to testify to the fact in case I would ever have need of proof one day that mental calibre could be so markedly altered by such a change in diet. The child herself felt impelled by her own ambitions to return to the less attractive diet.

I had long ago found that a reversal of symptoms could be secured in ten days, so it seemed important to persist with each experiment for that length of time, although improvement could be seen in three to four days. Or, if symptoms occurred- particularly in the period of half to three hours after a meal- to look at any food or substance that might have been introduced in the belief it was innocuous.

The most spectacular of these were-
a) Childrens' medicines in syrups. By the end of a course of medicine, the children would be wakeful, almost unmanageable, even violent. I checked and found the syrup base was glucose syrup.
b) Puffed wheat 'honey smacks'. The memory of the maniacal effect of these on my oldest daughter was one of the things that convinced me to attempt the gluten-free diet. I checked and found the word honey was misleading advertising. They were not coated with honey at all, but with glucose syrup.
c) Differential results in eating sweets. Some were worse in their effects than others. By diligent enquiry I found that there was not simply one glucose syrup, but a range identified as high or low maltose conversions. The maltose level could range as high as 60% or more. I identified the worst reactions as associated with the highest maltose levels.
d) Akta-vite in a chocolate tonic food like Ovaltine.

As the gluten-free diet seemed devoid of vitamins, I gave Akta-vite as a supplement. When the results seemed plainly adverse, I rang the Sydney office of Nicholas Pty. Ltd. to check on its contents to be told it contained no glucose syrup. So I persisted. But results continued adverse. I rang again. This time the Sydney office checked with head office in Melbourne. who confirmed my belief. Akta-vite was 55% crystalline glucose syrup. A very apologetic Sydney office brought me out a large gift box of their products. We had Radox baths for weeks on the strength of it.

Each one of these three examples was a blind trial of the validity of my suspicions. There were others. I became increasingly convinced that glucose syrup had beyond any doubt to be incriminated.

But reaction in general from professionals was sceptical. All starch is ultimately converted to glucose, they said, and they could not see that it mattered whether this conversion was initiated within, or without, the body. I did not ask the obvious question. Was there a difference between manufacturing glucose within the body by its endogenous enzyme systems, or ingesting quantities of free glucose or maltose in proportions higher than those freely occurring in nature? I did ask the other question that had begun to lurk in the back of my mind. Where do all the diabetics come from?

If the sceptics were right, and I was wrong, another question remained to be answered. What were the maltose levels in the

29

gluten-free diet we had been following? If they were lower than in normal diet, or even non-existent, this might explain our dramatic response on the coeliac diet compared with the one of which we had been so doubtful, the absence of gluten. As I have said before, we did not conform to the profile for gluten sensitivity except in some superficial resemblances. Was it possible we were not affected by gluten at all, but only by the carbohydrate of the whole wheat flour of which the glucose syrup was made?

I believed the answer must lie in the difference between whole wheat flour and cornflour. I resorted to ringing those obliging industrial chemists once more. Cornflour was the end product after gluten had been separated from carbohydrate. The maltose levels were insignificant. We had reduced them much as people remove lactose by removing milk from their diet. Hallelujah! An exciting new thought occured to me. If maltose was indeed the toxic factor in wheat, it might be possible to exploit the fact that it was one of the reducing sugars in the dynamics of digestion by dealing with it in some way other than the more drastic separation of starch from gluten, a way that would produce a more acceptable food than the coeliac cakes and bread with all the defects inevitable from a lack of gluten with its special leavening properties.

I rang the Bread Research Institute, and was lucky to be referred to a carbohydrate chemist there, one Dr. Zentner. He proved to be most courteous and open-minded to my theory (as had been true of many other industrial chemists). His answer was exciting, both in the scientific and the personal sense. Yes, it was possible to test the theory that maltose was the culprit, and not gluten, by leavening the bread long enough for all the maltose to be fermented away. How long would that take, I asked? At least six hours, he said. 'Surely all bread is fermented for that length of time,' I naively responded, remembering the old days when bread was made overnight in what was known as 'long' doughs.

No, he said, the good old days are gone. Bread is made in 'short doughs' with bread improvers, bread that is proved and out on the street in at most four hours, which means it is fermented for a very much shorter time, often only for one half to two hours. Part of the reason for this was that the 1945 Bread Act had required that bakers no longer worked two shifts, but completed their baking in one eight hour shift. This Act had provided a clear watershed between the old and the new.

His remarks provoked my memory at once. That year, 1945, was about the time when I became aware of a striking difference in my health. In my youth, we had eaten only white bread made by the old method, and not as much of it as the later generation. We had included a far greater variety of other starches in our diet, such as sago, tapioca, arrowroot, or cornflour. When I had switched to a wholemeal diet in the Womens College at Sydney University, my health had taken a downturn, and plunged to zero after I left College, as I increased the intake of wholemeal everything. This may have been due not only to shorter fermentation, but also the fact that fermentation is less effective or slower with wholemeal than white flour. The worse I became, the more health foods I ate under the twin delusions they would make me better, and help me to keep me slim.

Dr. Zentner's information plainly had enormous importance as it shifted our focus altogether from gluten to maltose, and offered an explanation as to why the coeliac diet had worked for us when we were not coeliacs. The next step was obvious- to restore wheat gluten to our diet as bread fermented for six hours, but not in any unfermented guise as in breakfast foods, biscuits, cakes etc. This would settle the gluten issue once and for all. But we would use white flour only as we were still doubtful about wholemeal for reasons we could not wholly explain.

The chemists at Fielders (now Goodman Fielders), who had been so helpful on the subject of glucose syrup, now arranged for their bakers to show me how to make and bake bread. The result was successful beyond my wildest expectation. The children had no behavioural or allergic symptoms so long as they only ate wheat when fermented. If they ate wheat that was not fermented, as happened when visiting or on school holidays, they would have minor lapses. These were no longer so important, provided they did not persist through a number of days. If they did there could be trouble, as for example when Rosalind, then aged eleven, went to National Fitness Camp and came back with dozens of hives from Weetbix, or Leone came back from riding camp with a burst blood vessel in her eye. She still has it, and it gets worse if she is tired, or off her diet.

Some of the fine details escape me now, but it has to be remembered I was not only pioneering a new theory with all its daily observations and extra work, but also had the responsibility of an ageing mother-in-law and father-in-law; all the usual alarms of family life- broken bones, infections, operations; and the customary chores of shopping, school commuting and functions.

31

Moreover I had to guard my inner fortitude to maintain the certainty of logic in the successive steps pursued.

Perhaps if I had not begun a Phd degree at this point, I would have made more careful notes, but then I needed the distraction to avoid becoming the world's greatest bore on a diet noone had ever heard of, nor could possibly understand. If you don't believe me, then try explaining to someone that you have a wheat intolerance which causes you to refuse cakes, biscuits, etc, but yet you are still eating bread. Or that you can eat one brand of ice-cream and not the rest. Except that I should add that a chemist or biochemist, who can instantly speak the necessary language, would understand. At that stage they were a courteous species that existed only on the telephone. And I talked to dozens, hours at a time, in order to make up my list so as to avoid the villainous glucose syrup lurking in drinks, ice-creams, sweets, and many other foods; or merely to confirm suspicions it was there. This lengthy chore was essential because foods were never labelled as to contents, but it had the advantage of enabling me to verify my instinctive findings all the time, and to learn the basics of food chemistry.

Looking back I was remarkably lucky that none of the children rebelled violently away from the rigours of the modified coeliac diet that I had now evolved in terms of the maltose theory, and my reasonably strict enforcement of it. This was surprising in view of some of my inconsistencies and changes, particularly on the question of associated glucose intake, leading me to experiment with diabetic foods and alternative sugars used by diabetics such as sorbitol and 'Sweetaddin'. In time I succeeded in arriving at a diet which removed all obvious symptoms, and almost all signs of derangement of metabolism, leaving only a marginal susceptibility.

I had done this by

a) excluding all known sources of 'added' glucose syrup in foods, e.g. icecreams, sweets, and drinks.

b) excluding the grains of wheat, rye, oats, and barley, unless fermented in a 'long dough' bread, preferring the grains of rice and corn.

However the logic of this had inherent problems of proof, of which I was well aware. This was to prevent me pushing the hypothesis of 'maltose' intolerance for some years to come.

a) If I argued that maltose was the offending factor in the reducing sugars of grains, and it was all but removed with adequate fermentation, this did not seem to make much sense in terms of other starches like potatoes or corn from which maltose could be

produced, unless there were other corollary factors.
b) If I argued that maltose alone was involved, how could I explain
   reactions from grapes (dried or fresh), or wine? Or from fruit
   juice, jam, or sugared fruit where initial sucrose had reduced into
   component glucose and fructose?

   The only possible factor that seemed to link all three was
glucose itself. I tested this theory with several doctors, including
my friend, Dr. Gordon Archer, Director of the Blood Bank, who had
been very helpful on the subject of maltose and allergy in general.
They all, albeit politely, laughed me out of court. How could you
possibly be allergic to your own blood sugar, they cried? And yet,
and yet, could they possibly be wrong, could excess even facilitate
allergy? The thought niggled for the next twenty years. It would
have niggled more, if I had realised then just how high the levels
of 'glucose' were in glucose syrup, which I wrongly believed then to
be insignificantly small. On this hypothesis, I still regarded
maltose as the sole villain, and, moreover, had other reasons for
thinking so.

   There was the fact that my oldest daughter had been given
a dose of maltose in the childrens' ward in a Melbourne hospital on
the last day of her stay there for exhaustive tests with both
herself and her sister for sucrose and fructose intolerance, and as I
supposed for maltose intolerance. But the eleven needles Rosalind
had to tolerate, and the biopsy Leone had to suffer, were only for
sucrose and fructose. The doctors concerned, who took no case
history, nor made any appointment with me, only gave Rosalind a
token dose of maltose on the last day. They took no samples, made
no observations or report, and discharged her from the hospital
shortly after. She had a violent muscular spasm half an hour after
ingesting the maltose, knocking the bedside table over; vomited
badly that night; and developed severe bronchitis that lasted two
days.

   Obviously those doctors did not consider my maltose theory
should be taken seriously. Certainly they did not consult me at any
time, nor tell me anything about results. They were invisible. As
had often been my experience, mothers were not supposed to know
anything. In my case, where I had made some important
observations, it was an insult I must bear. It was clearly not worth
my time, or effort, to report on what happened after Rosalind had
left the hospital.

   I was aware by this time that a nephew, Michael, was
affected. My association with him began at the point where he

33

had systematically failed in medicine and science at the University. When his father, my brother Alan, was deploring the fact, I said, 'are you sure he hasn't got the same thing as my children?' Alan encouraged Michael to talk to me when he came down to begin a Veterinary Science course at Sydney University. In fact, he stayed with me for some weeks in first term.

Michael's own account was of an increasingly erratic, even bizarre, response to his college environment, with a disrupted ability to concentrate. This latter problem had been familiar to me during my late teens and early twenties, causing a decline in my ability to keep my attention on the text of a lecture for any length of time. Michael adopted our diet so far as he could do so with sufficient success to pass through Veterinary Science, arguably one of the most difficult of all University courses.

During his first year at Sydney University, he began to dent my profound ignorance of enzyme systems (part of his course of study). As a result, I believed at the time that the enzymes, maltase and invertase, were interchangeable, and tried to adopt the practice of allowing the very occasional deviation from the diet only when wheat and sucrose were not together, e.g. a pizza would be better than a cake. Whether I was right, or clutching at straws, remains an open question, as I did not keep a daily diary. But it seemed to work at the time as a means of offering the children a bonus day, perhaps because this usually meant the child was consuming a rounded item of food rather than an ice-block or starch-oriented item.

In general the system I had devised worked well enough. However, I was not as yet totally convinced I had the right answer. I had not yet resolved minor paradoxes. For example, some of the symptoms were similar to those of coeliacs, such as a tendency to low blood calcium levels, to iron or folic acid deficiency, and ready bruising of the skin. Therefore I was reluctant to evangelise, or give advice. Even if I had, I doubt if people would have listened. They either took me for a diet freak, or simply could not follow what I was talking about. Most of them had an abysmal knowledge of the simplest chemistry, botany, or even their own physiology.

I was also aware by now that not only one of my nephews, but also an older and a younger sister were affected. Both had virtually stopped eating wheat in any quantity, if at all, some years before, and one of the two avoided dairy products as well- a choice that had nothing to do with me.

During these years, I was in correspondence with people overseas for a time, through whom I learnt that coeliacs, and other wheat allergics, responded to extra Vitamin C and certain B vitamins. It was a case of people who knew people who knew, or other frustrated parents. Some of them were what my children would call 'way out'. I dabbled with diabetic foods, and found many similarities in the pattern of our eating to those of diabetics, except that we had a much wider margin of tolerance in starch levels.

My children were growing up, and their sensitivity did not seem to be quite so great once the major spurts of growth and teething were over. I was more or less able to maintain the diet, gradually less rather than more as I became involved with researching a PhD, and then in running theatres. The latter became a trap, as the public theatre had a lolly bar, and my children used to clamour to serve the sweets sometimes, sampling the goods themselves. I daresay they were roughly following the principles they had learned, whenever they were away from home, but as they got older I lost track of their eating habits. As I had leaned heavily on them in childhood I did not wish to pursue them later because it was undoubtedly true that parents could create more of a problem pushing a special diet, than the diet itself. They had to decide for themselves whether they needed to maintain the diet in adult life, or whether they could now subsist on normal diet.

The one who continued to have a real problem was my third daughter, Eloise. She had always struggled in the school system from her earliest days in infant school. Certain aspects of this struggle did not appear entirely diet-related at that time- for example with flash cards and cuisinaire rods which gave her trouble in early learning, and later with abstract vocabulary and metaphor, which gave her trouble with compulsory subjects like English literature in late primary and early high school. At this date I only knew of the effect of diet in causing dislocation of thought and concentration. I had not realised how it could create learning difficulties in other ways. In first year high school, a psychologist tested her, and found she could read the text, but could not precis their meaning at the end of a page. In other words, she had a very deceptive learning profile.

When Eloise was floundering, mid-high school, her general practitioner at last decided to drop any psychological stress diagnosis, and sent her to a specialist, Dr. Steinbeck, who concluded from her history that she had temporal lobe epilepsy, and for a time she was treated in those terms. With hindsight, of course, the symptoms could just as easily have been those of hypoglycaemia, because hypoglycaemia can cause mild epileptiform seizures and other symptoms manifest in her, but in those days no doctors seemed to be as aware of that possibility as the doctors of a generation earlier.

Now that the child concerned is an adult with a child herself, she is somewhat judgmental of that period in her life. She does not yet realise the stress a parent in my predicament may suffer, which has been mentioned to a certain extent in this story. However she is quite definite about one thing today. She would have finished school if she had not been eating wheat.

A recent check with the veterinary science nephew was interesting. He had abandoned his diet on graduation, and returned to a modified normal diet. Like many wheat allergics said to have surmounted the propensity, he had had an optimum period. Then, according to his account, he began to suffer a decline in health. When I asked him why he had not made more concerted efforts to correct the situation, he said he was like an alcoholic pretending that the very thing that did most harm was harmless, because he could not find the willpower or the way to give up wheat. He began to follow my renewed dialogue with experts with interest and comments of his own, e.g. when dogs had allergies, he fed them rice.

As time passed, the family began to ask questions. Leone about her husband, for example. Matthew had had trouble with his sinuses all his life. Well my sinuses had cleared up forever on our low gluten diet. Let him try. He did. They did. Matthew and Leone religiously made their own bread for some years while they were in London, and now secure it regularly from a Sydney baker by the month.

By 1981 my children began to produce grandchildren. Rosalind had Emily that year, and Leone had Harriet not long after, followed by Rebecca two years later. In 1985, Vivian had Alexander. In 1987, Rosalind had Mark, and in this year of writing Eloise had Christian and Vivian a second boy, Breton.

The first five of these children began to present with problems. The last two were still too young to say. Their problems forced me into two courses of action:
a) voluntary- checking back on everything I knew to find answers to questions as yet unanswered.
b) involuntary- two short series on the identification of sugars; and

one that lasted years involving bread a baker made for us, but not, as it transpired, to the formula we had prescribed.

Or should I say that my children, particularly my oldest daughter, Rosalind, egged me on, which I suppose was inevitable, because I was the only one with the faintest idea of what it was all about. I was the one who had talked to dozens of chemists twenty years before, and had come to know the technicalities. But their questions made it clear that I did not understand the subject adequately. For example, were malt and maltose equally suspect? Was corn likely to be a problem because glucose syrup was manufactured from corn as well as wheat? And so on.

It was no longer simply good enough to say 'Read the labels on the products', which by now were on all products, or to say 'Avoid any foods that are labelled 'glucose syrup'. Though, by the way, such an instruction would have been a trap for young players, as some products such as medications simply said 'sugar syrup' or 'sugar free', when in fact they contained glucose syrup. I had to resolve the inherent paradoxes I have already mentioned. I had to look for some simpler proposition that would bind the elements together. Otherwise how on earth could I do as they asked and 'Write it all down in case something happens to you' (nice thought!), if I could not explain it with absolute clarity to myself?

I embarked on the final stages of this rocky road roughly from 1984-9 intermittently at first, then with much heavier involvement 1986-9.

THE GRANDCHILDREN

The problems of Emily were not spectacular at first. Born in 1981, she managed well enough on 'Carnation' tinned milk, after being weaned at several months' old. As her mother was on the staff of Macquarie University, she was in a nursery there, eating ordinary bread. She developed eczema on both legs at fourteen months.

She did not develop asthma until she was three, after dusty old underfelt was thrown from a flat upstairs down to the level where she lived. During the two years after the first onset of her asthma, it was not so bad as it became after she was five years old. During that period she was having a hot meal every midday in the winter, and therefore less commercial bread. A staff member of the Woollahra Municipal Kindergarten, Margaret Cloonan, noticed she was better behaved and less bad tempered when she was not eating sandwiches than when she was.

When Emily started school at five years of age, she began to have sandwiches every day. Her colour was poor, her eyes swollen and dark underneath. She was fidgety, irritable, and argumentative, particularly later in the day or when tired. She was capable of oddity and truculence. Now Rosalind had noticed on several occasions that Emily reacted severely to various products. She rang the chemist of the pharmaceutical company which manufactured Amoxil anti-biotics after a particularly bad reaction to Amoxil syrup, given over a week three times a day. The same was true of Pentavite vitamin tablets.

Although maltose dextrins were present only in a minute amount, they precipitated Emily into using Ventolin for her asthma. She was also unreasonable, tearful, prone to backtalk, and suffered from dilated eyes. I had noticed the same reactions in Rosalind when a child, though not necessarily with penicillin products. Rosalind was to find that Emily's younger brother, Mark, repeated the pattern.

When he developed an asthma-like cough after a course of syrup for a middle ear infection, and ended up at childrens' casualty at the Prince of Wales Hospital on ventilan, she suspected the syrup as the cause, as Emily had become very irritable on the chewable version of the same medication. She rang the drug company that marketed that particular product. They confirmed her suspicions. Rosalind has devised a way of overcoming the problem. When she visits a doctor with the children, she refuses to accept a prescription for any medication either in syrup or tablet form, as usually given children, but requires an adult prescription. She then empties the contents, and, on doctor's instructions, gives half the given dose in a little jam, or juice. Her youngest sister has found it necessary to follow the same formula with her son, Alexander.

The reason why drug companies began to use maltose dextrins as a base for medicine instead of the old, familiar sugar, was clamour about the effect of sugar in causing dental caries in children. But those people, who blithely labelled their medicines "sugar-free", had no thought for behaviour problems.

Emily also suffered a bad reaction after a Mintie Hunt. When Rosalind told me of this, I reminded her that her sister Eloise's adverse reactions to Minties had begun my own long maltose hunt so many years ago, and caused me to ring Mr. Jarman at Sweetacres. The incident was a useful reminder to maintain the caution usually observed in doling sweets out to these children.

Emily had also had problems with 'Poppa' pre-packed fruit juices popular among children. They would cause irritability and a runny nose. The only drink that proved acceptable was unsweetened pineapple. This later proved the case with Alexander and Mark.

Even with all precautions to limit maltose/glucose intake, Emily's asthma was so bad by Xmas 1987 she was wheezing every night, and had been to hospital casualty more than once. Her daily dependence on Ventolin for serious breathing problems had become so great, Rosalind was very worried. What should she do? I suggested there was only one way, the hard way. No modified diet with shop bread, not even the so-claimed 'long' dough I had persuaded a local baker to make (other wheat products were limited). A reduced level of fruit juices (always very liberal by old-fashioned standards). A strict supervision to exclude maltose. A serious adherence to the coeliac diet I had once used to stabilise herself.

If her problem was a severe maltose problem, there should be a dramatic improvement in six weeks. And, above all, arguments from the Asthma Council literature about stress, pollen, dust mites, and pollution to be put aside, so as to observe the child more clearly without complication. My reason for urging this was that these factors, although aggravating if the original irritant was present, had ultimately only proved secondary in my case. All sensitivity to them cleared up the moment the primary factor was removed.

In earlier days, I had been prostrated with hay fever for days by shaken carpets, perfume, privet or wattle blossom, to mention only a few before my diet changed. Once the primary factor was gone, none of these factors could provoke so much as a sniffle.

Emily was now of an age and intelligence where it was possible to secure her co-operation (a little younger than her mother when I began withdrawal experiments). She had found her asthma attacks very distressing, and was enthusiastic about relief.

I was in England when Emily passed the three weeks specified, and she was not yet quite free of asthma. Rosalind began to get downhearted, and to say the Asthma Council must be right, that other factors must also be operative. I asked her to perservere a little longer, an urging which proved justified. Emily's asthma disappeared in four weeks. She was overjoyed, and only too willing to accede to the differential problems of her diet.

At first Rosalind made gluten-free bread with a Basco bread mix from health food shops. She also made pastries, cakes and biscuits with their other mixes. After some months she rang me to ask me whether I could find out somewhere if the formula for any of these mixes had changed. She had begun to have trouble again. I asked her if she thought there was any difference between the four mixes she nominated- bread, cake, pie and biscuit. She nominated two, the pastry and the biscuit mix. I looked at the formula, and thought the problem must lie in the emulsifiers stated as present in these two. I tracked these emulsifiers back to Brisbane. They were malto-dextrins, recently introduced to prevent lumpiness in the mixes (a tendency with the soya flour). Once again, industry's leading concern was to satisfy consumer demand for appearance in product, and ease of handling. And once again we were victim to the crowd-pleasing of the new technology.

Then, as these bread mixes were very expensive, I made enquiries to see if it was possible to buy a gluten-free mix in bulk. I found that Mauri Brothers and Thompson had fifty kilo bags, marketed as gluten-free, based on a formula they said the Coeliac Society had recommended. Full of enthusiasm, I bought two gigantic bags. The mix was a disaster. Emily was irritable and had asthma. Again it was a case of tracking down the ingredients from warehouse to laboratory. The formula seemed impeccable at first glance- cornflour, raising agents, and milk powder. Nothing else, not even soya flour. As Mauri Brothers manufactured cornflour, I presumed it was as blameless as cornflour we had used in the past. I rang Rosalind back and said so, traversing the diet she gave Emily for other possible causes. The days passed. She insisted the mix was the cause of the trouble, as indeed it proved to be. When she withdrew it from Emily's diet, she got better.

I rang Mauri Brothers, and was surprised when I learned the actual proportions of the ingredients of the gluten-free mix. Some twenty five percent was skimmed milk powder, and seven percent pregelatinised starch. I was horrified that the fraction of milk powder was so high. Doubt still hung over our capacity to handle milk in any quantity. But more important, doubt existed more over certain types of manufactured milk products, such as long-life milks, which were preserved by superheating (to be mentioned in relation to my other grandchildren). Was powdered milk also a superheated milk? I rang Petersville, manufacturers of the milk powder. Did the milk powder have to be superheated in its manufacture? The answer was yes, which raised yet more questions. Was the adverse effect due to the high level of lactose, or to possible distortion of protein, or both? The first question led me to a detailed consideration of the frequency of lactose intolerance among humans, and the chance we shared in this. The second uncovered a debate among biochemists as to whether protein changed or not, which still stands undecided.

There was also the question of pregelatinised starch. Did the processes involved in its manufacture change the starch in some undesirable way? The accounts I could find were occupied with explaining the virtues of pregelatinisation in improving product, not its potential vices. Perhaps there are none. But this question still remains adjourned.

In the upshot, Rosalind stopped using the mix, and I was left with two large bags on my hands. Mauri Brothers took one bag back, but I still have the other, and use it experimentally from time to time to see if it affects me. I would say it does if used daily. I have noticed similar problems with a gluten-free bread mix sold in supermarkets in Ireland (though it has added soya flour to complicate any enquiry into its effect).

A year later I spoke to a Mr. Johnston at Goodman Fielders to make absolutely sure I was correct in believing that cornflour was free of residual maltose whether the cornflour came from wheat or corn, before completing this record. He said it was.

During this year, Rosalind had been obliged to make up all her own mixtures. Occasional crises still occurred, as when Emily ate a large quantity of cornflake cookies smothered in honey. It seemed she could eat honey when it was uncooked, but not when it was cooked. Rosalind further refined Emily's diet by reducing milk to the amount required for baking. Altogether her asthma was vastly improved. She only needed her ventilan intermittently when she got wheezy from time to time, especially when under bodily stress through spurts of growth etc, but not in the chronic way as before.

Rosalind found that any problems remaining were minor. Sometimes extended use of rice flour (white without bran) made her nose irritable. But in general, rice flour was much more easily digested than wheat, barley, oats or rye. Emily remains remarkably free of asthma other than in exceptional circumstances, such as consumption of two packets of cough lozenges, and participation in a long fun run.

Rosalind's son, Mark, was six years younger than Emily when he was born. He was gradually weaned at nine months. His solid diet was already gluten free, according to the standard practice in infant welfare at present which excludes wheat until one year of age on the grounds the immune response which characterises coeliac disease is less likely to occur. Therefore, when he started on formula milks, and problems began to occur, it was clear the source of the trouble could not be gluten. Rosalind tested some seven different brands in all during a rather dementing trial period. In each case, a reaction developed within a week. In fact, Infasoy over a month or so produced the asthma-like cough she knew so well from Emily.

In searching for any factor linking the brands, it seemed the common denominator must be 'corn' syrup. Therefore she discarded any formulae which listed 'corn syrup' on its contents. Having reached that conclusion, she was intrigued to have it corroborated by an independent observation made to her by Sister Pam Day of the Double Bay Health Centre that corn syrup caused some people a lot of difficulty. In all, Rosalind tried some seven different brands with Mark, every one of which produced varying degrees of irritability and coughing. 'Nan' was worse than the others, causing him to be very cross, wakeful, and scream inconsolably, even to pass to a minor seizure state. He would cry intensely, and be absolutely inconsolable. If he was picked up, he would arch his back and be very stiff. The episode would pass off after a while, but recur several times in a night. She had to discard the idea of using a lactose-free formula (lactose being converted to its component galactose and glucose) as this also caused reactions.

I had hopes of Infasoy, a soya bean substitute, which had worked for the second daughter of my second daughter, Leone, some four years before (and a similar product for my fourth daughter some years before). But these hopes proved unjustified. He reacted badly yet once again. I checked back with the company who made it to ask the all-important question. Had any component of this soy-milk formula been changed in the past four years since Rebecca had had it? The answer was yes. They had substituted glucose syrup for sucrose to create a product less threatening to dental caries. Once more the horror of creeping glucose syrup had caught up with us all, this time in the name of benefit to mankind. And once more we had had an inadvertent blind trial of our conviction of the malign effect of glucose syrup.

In the end, Rosalind had to retreat back to one of the first baby milk formulae she had tried as the only one that was tolerable, namely S26, and that only in the infant formula even until he was two years old, when Rosalind had to abandon it altogether. The S26 Progress was definitely not satisfactory. One of the least tolerable effects was the child's tendency to unsettled sleep through the night. One of the worst experiences Rosalind had in this regard was when Mark was ten months old. She had taken him to New Zealand, and, while there, had run out of S26. She bought a formula called SMA Gold Cap, which had S26 listed underneath, which suggested that it was the same formula. As a result, he woke hourly through the night.

Much more recently, her younger sister, Eloise, complained of her ten month old son's wakefulness at night, and showed her the same tin as had caused similar trouble. She too now uses S26. An interesting point about the S26 formula was that it contained whey, and therefore reasonably high levels of lactose. She felt he had to continue on some breastmilk substitute until he was older, despite reservations she or I had about its effect on the child, such as what I call the dynamo effect (not the same as 'hyperactivity') and frequent motions. As his maltose levels were very low, an accentuation of difficult behaviour was puzzling at first- namely irritability, arching back, inconsolable crying- either when she called for him at the infant nursery, or in the middle of the night (these episodes were self-limiting for about 10-20 minutes).

Rosalind realised finally that Mark's problem was related to the Sunburst 'reconstituted' orange juice he was having twice a day in the nursery. It was labelled only 'sugar syrup', and I could not elucidate what that meant when speaking to the manufacturer; nor learn whether the rind was crushed with the orange in order to make it, which might have contributed citral to the drink. The same happened in the one-year-old nursery. Nose streaming, crying etc., although the juice was only used sometimes. In his second year, when the orange juice was the only juice used, the problem was much more exaggerated. Rosalind solved it by changing back to the practice she had adopted in the nursery. She supplied Mark's own juice for him- unsweetened pineapple juice. These days his adverse reactions are likely to be limited to occasional biting rather than screaming fits lying on the ground.

In this context, it is worth noting that his father was irritable and moody when he was drinking beer every day, and developed a chronic sinus. He never has more beer now than the occasional social drink, which clearly causes his sinuses to swell, as he snores thereafter. And high malt beers like Guiness are much worse offenders in this than the light beers. His sinuses also flare up after the occasional bread or cake 'binge'.

Mercifully, my second daughter did not seem to have such severe problems with her two daughters. They seemed to manage on a modified low maltose diet, and making their own 'long dough' bread while in London, changing to the bakery bread specially made by a baker at Bondi Junction when they became too busy to make their own. Though they were not altogether free of what I would have considered symptoms, they did not develop the frank allergic reaction of their cousins, and were less severely affected than Rosalind's children with fluctuations of temperament. As I saw less of them than the other grandchildren, it was harder to monitor them. But Leone did mention wakefulness, anxiety, clinging, stubborn spells, timidity, etc. she did not, however, mention any digestive problems until recently when the oldest, Harriet, began to complain of headaches, and the youngest, Rebecca, of both headaches and stomach cramps. Their mother, my second daughter, Leone, also spoke of her own intolerance to instant coffee, packet soups (which use malto-dextrins) and powdered milk (which incriminates lactose). But I would not have expected them to be free of symptoms altogether, as their diet was more relaxed than that of the other two families of grandchildren in relation to unfermented wheat, eating pastas, spaghetti, and pizzas which are forbidden in my diet. For that reason, I took far too long to realise something was amiss with the commercial bread we all obtained from Bondi Junction, but which neither myself nor my eldest daughter ate any longer.

I continued to think of it as being preferable to commercial bread, particularly after an incident which proved Rebecca's tolerance was far better on the Bondi Junction bread than ordinary shop bread. Leone had resorted to commercial bread during a change-over from an old freezer to a new frig-freezer. The deterioration in Rebecca's personality and appetite was conspicuous, and she became much harder to manage. Leone reverted to using the specially-made bread. However, as time wore on this too became suspect. Both children were suffering quite frequent headaches and Rebecca was constantly complaining of stomach cramps. I still put these problems down to the cumulative effect of sources of unfermented wheat in their diet due to the fact a 'nanny' was doing the cooking, which made it harder to sustain a difficult diet. Then suddenly I had reason to know I was wrong. The Bondi Junction bread should have been suspect all along, as I will explain in the story of the son of my fourth daughter, Alexander, their younger cousin.

Alexander's story is important, because he is one of the best subjects to observe of us all. He, like Christian and Mark, was on S26 when weaned at about nine months, but was very restless and wakeful. He could not tolerate whole milk, or soymilk, and was quite uncontrollable on UHT or long-life milk at the end of a week. His reaction to the latter was as if he were on a superhigh-uncontrollable, running everywhere, kicking, bashing, refusing to go to sleep, jumping, and having hysterical screaming fits. He could only tolerate goat's milk in a powdered brand from New Zealand.

Vivian learnt quite early that his reaction to 'Poppa' juice was the same as Mark's. He would become very active, out of control and odd in his behaviour, or lie down on the floor in hysterical kicking tantrums. Such behaviour was clearly abnormal, as he had a very calm, stable personality if not exposed to the wrong food.

Like Emily, Alexander had a full hot meal in the middle of the day during his nursery days, and continued to do so in Canberra, when he began to attend kindergarten there. He was being given a tiny portion of wholemeal or brown bread once a day, but otherwise he was not eating bread at other meals. He was capable of tolerating a small intake of wheat in the odd meal on occasional days. But when Vivian reintroduced one or two glasses of milk for the first time since he was a baby, after a build up of a week or so,

45

he was in trouble all the time. When he was being obnoxious, he would get the staring or squiffy eyes I remembered from my oldest daughter when young. Vivian pulled him back to milk on cereals only, and his bad behaviour disappeared.

At first Vivian struggled with the usual alternatives to bread- rice cakes and biscuits and so on. But eventually, on my suggestion, she found a baker who would make her a 'long dough' solely with yeast in a five hour fermentation. No bread improvers with their malt flour. This worked like a dream, and once more proved that the resolution lay in removing the maltose, and not the gluten, as Vivian also found with other products like ice-creams, lollies. Sometimes she said she would 'goof' and give him something like Devon sausage without realising it could have the enemy lurking in the filling along with the meat, with the same dire results. She also found he fared badly on supermarket juices, except for pineapple juice.

At this point when Alexander's diet was well under control, Vivian moved back to Sydney; a move which led to a quite unscheduled revelation. She no longer had a source of supply for her bread, but was able to get a supply of Bondi Junction bread from her sister, Leone, who happened to be going on holiday. At the end of a week, Vivian rang me in tears. Within seven days on this bread, Alexander had become quite bizarre and maniacal. He made silly, repetitive tongue movements, booed and screamed for attention, laughed uncontrollably, talked non-stop, jumped in a frenzied manner, and pursued his mother with verbal abuse e.g. 'You stupid mum. How dare you go out of the room when I am not looking.' And so on, and so on. His normal personality was exaggerated to an extreme. For example, if he kissed his mother or the baby, he would kiss them forcefully and repeatedly. And by the seventh day, the abnormal behaviour was day-long. It was similar to behaviour exhibited on glucose syrup lollies, but worse.

I had made soothing noises when Vivian rang me up midweek and asked questions about other possible sources of trouble. But by week's end, she was begging me to go up to the baker and find out whether there was anything else about the bread. In the end, I agreed, remembering that Rosalind had said Emily had found that same bread intolerable after a somewhat longer trial, begetting asthma rather than the severe behaviour disorder that Alexander exhibited.

However, I was still puzzled. I had often picked up the batches of bread for the children, and questioned the baker at

46

Bondi Junction when Rosalind was beginning to have doubts. How was he making it? With yeast, he said. How long was he fermenting it? For three or more hours he said. I had had difficulty imbuing him with the importance of fermenting it for longer, and now thought Alexander's trouble might be due to the shorter fermentation of this bread compared to his Canberra bread. I was wrong, at least in part.

'Can you tell me exactly how you are making the bread?' I asked the baker who had always been so obliging. I say this advisedly, as baking special batches like ours is always disruptive to business. I then explained why I was asking the question. I was absolutely amazed to learn that he had always been adding bread improver, or 'Bakerine' as it is known, because, he said, the bread had not risen adequately with yeast alone. I was horrified. 'How much?' I asked. 'Only a very small amount,' he said apologetically, having seen the look on my face. 'What is a small amount?' I demanded. Only two tablespoons to over 40 loaves.

Here was the explanation of problems with all the children, that 'very small amount' of bakerine consumed consistently. I felt mortified that my daughters had relied on me, had had trouble, and I had taken so long to elucidate the cause. But first I had to be sure it was the cause. I rang the baker again for the name of the type of 'Bakerine' he used. Three telephone calls later I was speaking to Louise Sampson of Mauri Brothers and Thompson, the same lady who had given me the formula of the gluten free bread mix, to ask this time for the formula of the 'Bakerine'. Her answer was puzzling at first. Wheat flour, and chemicals, which she said firmly were approved by the National Medical and Research Council. Wheat flour? I came off the phone puzzled.

Suddenly Louise Sampson rang back, saying 'There's someone here would like to speak to you, who says it is the malted flour that is causing your trouble. Malted? She had not mentioned that, which goes to show how ingredient lists can sometimes be deceptive. It was Dr. Zentner, the very man who first suggested I should make bread with yeast and ferment it for six hours so many years ago at the Bread Research Institute. I was delighted. The wheel had come full circle. I could thank him for the difference he had made in my life, and was able to tell him so and what had happened since I last spoke to him. I could explain how people had shaken my faith in my own theory, so I had more recently been sidetracked into re-examining gluten and other possibilities just to make sure my theory could not be dislodged on other grounds.

47

But first I had to have an answer to the main point that had always made me doubt my own hypothesis. Could very small quantities of maltose cause all that trouble? Of course, he confirmed, almost exploding at the other end of the phone, maltose is a very powerful catalyst. That is why it is used in the bread industry- to create more and more maltose as the bread leavens. Therefore you must ensure a long fermentation until all the maltose is consumed, if you are deficient in maltase enzymes to deal with that maltose. He made no bones about it. A product of the natural dynamics of a common food could be as inimical as any of the artificial products of food engineering. He was also able to affirm that no matter how, or where, the malt appeared, whether as flavouring on breakfast cereals, in beer, or anywhere else, it made no difference. It should be excluded. And yet strangely enough, we had found 'Rice Bubbles', although malted, passable; a fact which had always made we wonder if other auxiliary factors were not involved in our problem.

In order to make absolutely sure the bakerine was the source of trouble- asthma, headaches, cramps, temperament- I asked the baker to make me a batch of bread without any bakerine; an exercise in which he was not proficient. The first batch of ten loaves were rather flat, but worked well enough with Alexander, and even little Mark (now two), who had been refusing the bread substitutes that made him different from the other children. The next batch was poor in quality, flat with a heavy crust. Despite its overshort fermentation of four hours, the children did not have the same overt symptoms as with the bread that had been leavened with the aid of 'Bakerine' or bread improver. I rang the head baker at the Bread Research Institute to ask him what was wrong. He said it sounded like a 'green dough', which could be due to the use of a high gluten flour. However, on a second phone conversation, he gave me a recipe he had worked out, and said that it would not matter if high gluten flour were used. I asked our baker to make a batch with this recipe. This time he left the dough to prove for five hours, and the result was better; but it was not as good as that from the batch of another baker I had found in my desperation to get back to the same perfect result as I had had when I used to make the six hour doughs on Dr. Zentner's formula.

This baker was an old-timer in a small business, willing to bake bread to an individual order such as ours, which no commercial bakery would contemplate for a moment. This baker ran us a trial batch made in the way he had learnt in his youth. He made it in two shifts- mixed at night with a small amount of yeast, left to prove all night, then punched down, tinned, left to rise, and finally baked next morning. Vivian is ecstatic. Alexander is an angel, she says. We are all ecstatic. I hope the baker is. He is probably breaking the Bread Act to do it.

During these two intensive years, 1987-9, when my children had independently made their own observations, and come to test, and verify, my conclusions for themselves as correct, fate had decreed that I should have the excellent good fortune to move into the University arena and to expose our theories to an even more rigorous test in the scientific world.

In these years of revival of the whole maltose question, fate determined that I should meet Professor Fraser, Professor of Animal Husbandry at Sydney University, or rather first it decreed that I was appointed to the Senate of the University of Sydney by the State Government of the day (in July 1987). So it happened that I was sent an invitation to inspect the Veterinary Science Farms at Camden, and went in the belief I should be trying to bridge the gaping areas of my scientific ignorance. I had no idea that a meeting with Professor Fraser awaited me, one which was about to change everything and to make far more sense out of the diet puzzles that hung over the family.

I did not speak to Professor Fraser until late in the day, and then primarily from my growing concern that the highly qualified staff of the faculty had given their time to inform a Senate of which only five had bothered to turn up, or take more than a limited interest. I asked Professor Fraser what his role was. He answered that he was a biochemist who was Professor of Animal Husbandry. I hailed him with an enthusiasm that may have surprised him. 'I have always wanted a chance to talk to one.' I mentioned my growing concern at the increasing emphasis in diet on wholemeal, and the attendant problem of phytic acid mentioned in baby booklets issued by the Health Department when my children were young. And so our acquaintance went on from there. His pleasant, friendly manner encouraged me to venture on the dread subject of carbohydrate intolerance, and I began to learn just how open-minded he was, and, in the months that followed, to understand that this was the hall-mark of biochemists who had made such brilliant advances in the previous decade.

Professor Fraser, it appeared, had worked on Vitamin D in Cambridge, and on the cause of rickets in Asian children in London, for which he was awarded a prize by the Rank Foundation. He had identified the rickets as due to the shift in the original diet of their homeland to a wholesale consumption of chappatis made of unleavened wheat, which had affected their calcium metabolism leading to the bone affectation of rickets.

I had long been aware of the original work of Mellanby in 1924, when he identified an unknown factor in the carbohydrate of oats as causing rickets. I had wondered at the time if the leg cramps my children suffered, before I removed maltose from the diet, were

50

involved with some problem of calcium malabsorption. I mentioned this to Professor Fraser, and provoked what I interpreted as mild interest, although it may merely have been polite interest. Anyhow, I arranged to see him again without too much hope of the encounter leading anywhere. There had been too much superficial interest in the past from others.

I enlisted Dr. Mary-Lou Shiels to give me a more professional credential. I had too often been treated as outside the 'club' because I was not a doctor. I had come by the link with Dr. Shiels in as oddly accidental a way as my meeting with Professor Fraser some months before. I had had a lunch date with a mutual friend, and as Dr. Shiels was late for her appointment with this friend (a travel agent) we all ended up lunching together. I refused the bread. She asked why. For some strange reason, I did not give my standard reply 'wheat', but said maltose. She immediately cross-examined me at length. The reason for her interest, it transpired, was that she had more than hundred patients who had come up maltose positive in tests with Dr. MacLean of Clinical Assays. She had no diet that worked with them, and at that stage was inclined to agree with the allergy clinic at Royal Prince Alfred Hospital that the maltose finding was a 'false positive', which I thought very odd. I said, 'Then let me see the diet,' which she did. It was incomplete and inappropriate. The dietitians who devised it had not taken into account the effects of modern food technology in raising the percentage of maltose in modern diet well above old-fashioned levels. No wonder that diet had not worked.

Dr. Shiels assigned an assistant to up-date the list of foods I had prepared some years before by phoning around dozens of companies, and to prepare a diet in terms of my explanations. I felt this list betrayed a failure fully to understand my theoretical approach. It reinforced my conviction that some simpler approach was necessary to get my points across. If I could not expect trained doctors to understand, how much less could I expect laymen to do so? However, I must emphasise that Dr. Shiels, as an allergist, had helped me with some more professional terminology for my somewhat idiosyncratic postulates with her comments on the state of the art of the allergy industry. And she was very supportive. She took part in the first test Professor Fraser proposed after he had heard our story. He suggested selecting six people thought to be maltose intolerant, and testing them to see if any of the maltose was not fully metabolised, but was excreted in the urine. Four of those prepared to take part in the test were known to conform to our profile- Dr. Shiels herself, myself, my daughter Rosalind, and her daughter Emily. The fifth, a patient of Dr. Shiels, was quite unknown to me, but was presumably selected for the probability that she was the same. The sixth was my husband. He had never had a similar profile to ourselves, but had been on our diet for some months for no better reason that all means of dealing with his bouts of dizziness had failed and he was then ready to try anything. Surprisingly it worked, with the added bonus of making him feel more energetic and cheerful.

Professor Annison of the Department of Animal Husbandry of the University of Sydney was kind enough to carry out the analysis of the samples, which were taken after the ingestion of five grammes of maltose on a fasting stomach. The result was negative. None of the maltose was excreted in the urine. It was all metabolised. But in other ways the result was quite dramatic.

1. Myself. Faint tingling, slight whooziness and light-headedness within an hour. Pain in the sites of old shoulder and back injuries. Clumsiness. Weeping of eyes and yawning after twelve hours.

2. Frank. Swollen irritable eyes, and persisting slight headache and nausea that lasted from one and a half hours through to six hours.

3. Rosalind. Irritability, irritated veins, and motor incoordination. Ocular dysfunction lasting for half an hour at twelve hours. Effect lasted for days.

4. Emily. Sneezing, and effects on nose and throat. Slight cough (usually the prelude to asthma). Sent out of the class for talking for the first time.

5. I did not have a report in detail from Dr. Shiels. But she did say she had felt hungry and confused, and confessed to motor incoordination.

Professor Fraser decided to conduct another test. This time I was the only one to be tested. It would take the form of a blind trial with five grammes each of five different reducing sugars. I would not know which was which, as the small phials would merely carry an identifying letter. In this way, it would not be possible for me to know which was maltose, and which was not. If I invented symptoms to support my maltose theory, I would be caught out.

I decided to take these sugars three days apart on a fasting stomach under stable conditions- that is, no basic changes in size, content or time of meals. I would drink them in a small glass of apple juice to mask sweetness or lack of it (the Professor's addition, not mine). Three out of the five sugars caused symptoms. Each of the three caused different symptoms, but only one of those three produced symptoms that were noticeably different. Two gave no symptoms at all. I rang Professor Fraser in some excitement, yet with some misgiving because my credibility was on the line if I pointed in the wrong direction, declaring maltose to be benign after saying so firmly it was not.

'E' is the worst I said. Professor Fraser opened his sealed envelope, and made the fateful remark, 'Why that's glucose!' The one sugar supposed to give the least trouble to the human race had given me the most trouble. 'I can't help it. It gave me the most trouble,' I replied defensively, thinking at first I had condemned myself. 'Such a small amount,' he commented, asking what the symptoms were. Yawning, running eyes, motor incoordination, and an irresistible desire to sleep after five hours.

The other two sugars that had given symptoms, each different, were galactose (from the inversion of lactose in milk) causing pain in the back and acute insomnia, and maltose causing sore eyes, tinitis, and heavy snoring. The remaining two that had given no symptoms were sucrose and fructose, the two I had said for many years gave us no problems, though sucrose at least had long been considered deleterious by many people.

This test jogged my memory, a recollection of some abnormality in glucose tolerance tests given my two oldest daughters at the Childrens' Hospital, Camperdown, on referral of a pediatrician, Dr. Kate Winning. But I did not know the details, as I had not been allowed to be present, nor was told the results. I rang my second daughter, and asked her if she could remember what happened. She was only seven at the time. She instantly said yes. She had cried, and been unable to complete the word 'rabbit' in the given squares of a puzzle she was doing, which normally she could do perfectly well. Rosalind, she recalled, had become violent. Because the reaction was unusual, the nurses had asked the Professor of Pediatrics, Professor Stapleton, to come over but he had refused. No reason was given for his refusal.

Here we had the explanation of the children reacting against fruit juices, my husband feeling affected after three glasses of orange juice, my intolerance of large intakes of cooked fruits, jams, etc. At moments like these I felt a sense of defeat. It was difficult enough to argue maltose intolerance, without adding glucose intolerance in its own right as well; unless of course one were

53

simply to say our diet was basically a pre-diabetic diet, a statement that was half true.

It was plainly foolish to cry halleluljah on the basis of one test. The five sugar test must be repeated. We were agreed the test this time must be without the additional apple juice in case it had obscured the accuracy of the result. So I took delivery of the innocuous little white phials. This was the rock on which I might shipwreck. Some three weeks later, I carried out the experiment as before, when it proved possible to do it without fluctuations in routine. A fasting stomach. A stable diet. A free schedule with time to observe. But this time a sample per day.

So I began this second trial, this make or break second test, by which I felt I would stand or fall. It engendered an excitement so solitary, so esoteric, few would appreciate it. Believing Professor Fraser would try to fox me, I reversed the series and began with E. The series proved puzzling. This time I only had symptoms with two samples out of five. Where was the insomnia, the back pain of galactose? The snoring of maltose? Nothing. Three blanks out of five. What had gone wrong with my powers of observation? It was two days before I had the courage to ring Professor Fraser, and nominate the two sugars which had given reactions. Then I waited like Henny Penny for the sky to fall in.

'The ones you have picked are both glucose!' he said triumphantly. Bravo! I had done it again. And the other three were all sucrose. No wonder they were all blank. Sucrose had never troubled us as sucrose. Right again. I had not tried to invent symptoms for those three phials of sucrose. No falling in the trap which Professor Fraser so sensibly set. Elated beyond belief, I offered to do the tests again.

Now the hue and cry to research glucose was on in earnest to see just whether the finding about glucose per se must qualify my finding about maltose, as I had always placed the emphasis on maltose rather than glucose, thinking of glucose merely as an excess facilitating maltose intolerance, and not as causing any problems in its own right. I had always believed the amount of glucose in glucose syrup to be small. Just how much glucose was there in glucose syrup, now so widely added to processed foods? I was astounded to be told by a manager at Fielders Goodman that the fraction could be as high as forty to fifty per cent in some glucose syrups. This meant that food technology was raising the levels of glucose, as well as maltose, way beyond the intake to be expected in the diet of former generations. Why did this not raise any doubts anywhere? Were

54

all the experts satisfied with the explanation I had so often been told- that glucose cannot possibly be harmful as it is the very substance that fuels your body? We had always found otherwise. Were they right, or we?

Professor Fraser headed me towards the Badham Library, where I began to wallow in the wonderful world of biochemistry, thankful for photocopiers, abstracts, indices of abstracts, and computer searches.

There was a lot of material available on glucose in relation to diabetics. Much of this work applied to non-insulin dependent diabetics, and to people with impaired glucose tolerance, which could presumably apply to myself and my family. Its chief concern was to stabilise their glucose response to enable them to continue without insulin. But it also happened to apply to athletes.

Such studies were concerned with issues such as-
a) the selection of 'slow release' cereals such as lentils.
b) the daily organisation of intake of carbohydrate.
c) the type of intrinsic fats in cereals, e.g. oats compared to wheat.
d) the combination of carbohydrates with other foods.

I also kept a weather eye out for any abnormal effect noted from the intake of excess glucose. Almost at once I came across a paper in a published record of a symposium on glucose syrup held in 1972 (slanted at industry technology), which reported tests carried out at Guys Hospital, London, to compare the effect on two groups of 'normal' volunteers of both glucose and glucose syrup. The volunteers on glucose could not complete the course of glucose because of nausea and dizziness. Those on glucose syrup could. From this result, the Professor concluded that glucose syrup was benign because it caused less immediate ill effect than pure glucose. He made no comment on the significance of such overt adverse reactions to glucose that the test was discontinued, thinking perhaps the amount used in the tests would not be likely to be achieved in the normal daily diet. Yet there is every reason to suppose these days they are.

At this time, I was relying heavily on my daughters to understand the dynamics of food and digestion better in order to report reliably back to me. At first it was an uphill battle. They knew only absolutes. Wheat was wheat, milk was milk, and so on. They were not foods subject to changes outside and inside the body, being transformed by processes within the machinery of that body. Changes I must briefly define in case my terms baffle my readers, as much as they did my children at first.

55

Man cannot utilise solar energy directly for his own energy requirements. Plants can. Therefore man must eat the plants in order to convert that energy for his own use. The carbohydrate of these plants consists of families of saccharides. One family is of complex molecules known as polysaccharides, oligosaccharides, and disaccharides. The other is of simple molecules known as monosaccharides. The complex molecules of the first family must all be split in the upper digestive tract to the simple molecules of the second family by enzymes. Most of these enzymes are in the brush border membrane lining that upper digestive tract or small intestine, the interior of which is impervious to all but monosaccharides in a healthy person. However, the membrane may cease to function properly as a protective barrier against disaccharides and become permeable when the digestive process is disturbed as in coeliac disease. If disaccharides enter the bloodstream, disturbance of immune and other functions can result.

The synthesis of carbohydrate simply defined above is in fact so complex that it took thirty years to work out how the cycle of digestion, absorption and oxidation, that became known as the Krebs Cycle, was achieved- through hydrolysis of various enzymes, regulation of several hormones (including insulin), and the thirty reactions of oxidation.

In this daunting world of intricate biochemistry, I had focussed on just two disaccharides, maltose and lactose, and one monosaccharide, glucose. The end result of the first two is the same, namely glucose, except they are split to glucose in a different way. Maltose splits to the one monosaccharide, glucose, in the small intestine; lactose to two monosaccharides, glucose and galactose, the latter of which is converted to glucose in the liver.

Some of the most powerful enzymes involved in this starch digestion are alpha-amylase and beta-amylase of the saliva and the pancreas, the former being a hundred times more powerful than the latter. The amylases of the saliva initiate the breakdown of the starch to glucose, while the amylases of the pancreas complete the process. The glucose then enters the bloodstream through the lining of the small intestine causing a rise of glucose in the bloodstream. This rise is controlled by insulin released from the pancreas, which removes any excess to store it as glycogen in the 'bank' of the liver.

Since the problem of myself and my family was that our saccharide digestion did not function properly with loads of maltose (and peripherally lactose), I had always thought only in terms of an inadequacy of maltase and lactase enzymes, which convert maltose and lactose. I was preoccupied entirely with reducing maltose, maltose/glucose and glucose to the smaller loads with which our presumably low enzyme levels could cope to prevent 'malabsorption', as it was known.

I knew nothing at all about another threat of paramount importance to us- namely the effect of 'inhibitors' presen in plant foodstuffs on the amylases and other enzymes, ana mineral absorption. I was aghast as I realised this threat existed as much in my habits with food in the kitchen, as it did in food engineering in the factory. I could no longer join the chorus which claimed it was all the fault of food processing, and the addition of unnatural additives to food. For inhibitors were not additives. They were natural to the plants.

I happened on knowledge of these inhibitors accidentally in 1988, and pursued the subject intermittently with a horrified fascination for the next year. For a long time, it seemed a maze without an exit, until suddenly in trying to solve an almost irrelevant riddle, I found the way out to a very simple resolution of considerable importance to us, and perhaps even to others who do not necessarily suffer our drastic reactions to maltose.

PHYTIC ACID

While the ferment of dialogue was proceeding with my children, I went back twenty five years in my mind to get a grip on the original heart of the matter. I had found then that we could eat wheat when fermented for a long time, but only if white, not brown. We found bran indigestible. The identification of maltose as our problem had never really resolved the question as to why we found a difference between well-milled white flour from which the bran had been removed, and wholemeal from which it had not, if both were well-fermented with yeast.

Now I had been exposed to bran before my children were born to a far greater degree than they later were. The more my health had become a problem, the more I had eaten 'health' foods, such as whole grains including wheat germ and wheat bran, strongly advertised as the secret of 'keeping your bowels healthy'. I did not relate severe stomach cramps, vomiting attacks, and prostrate hayfever with brans, nor did doctors, who spoke of gastric infection, pollens and so on. I had no reason to withdraw whole unfermented wheat foods like 'Weetbix', 'Vitaweat' or wholemeal biscuits from my childrens' diet in their infant years; although I never exposed them to other foods popular in my day like wholemeal porridge. So they suffered, as I had done until I was lucky enough to see it was the very 'health' foods supposed to give me good health which in fact were giving me bad health.

The puzzle lingered in my mind over the years. Why did we have a far greater sensitivity to wholegrain flour than white refined flour devoid of bran? Was there some other factor in bran, creating a further impediment to our maltose/glucose intolerance which might throw some light on the problem? But I could not devise even the sketchiest answer, as I did not fully understand the difference between bran and starch at that time.

I certainly did not know that bran, the husk of cereals, is the smaller, and relatively indigestible fraction of carbohydrate, the rest being starch, the larger, easily digestible fraction that provides our daily energy. I was totally ignorant that the fibre of bran does not furnish energy, but bulk in diet; that it is not digested in the small intestine, as starch is, but in the large intestine that lies beyond where it is digested by the fermentation of bacteria. I did know it was promoted by doctors as valuable in diet because it offered the highest fraction of vitamins and minerals in the original grain, and components thought to decrease chloresterol in the blood.

By Christmas 1987, the promotion of bran, or fibre as it was now called, was so successful that it was almost impossible for us to find anything that was not wholegrain, even in the foods still available to us. White rice cakes, for example, disappeared off the shelves in favour of brown. Half the health sweet bars, which had proved reasonably acceptable, except when they contained glucose syrup, were now muesli bars. Restaurants or aeroplanes served only brown, or wholemeal, bread or rolls. When I insisted on white rolls with an economy class steward on Qantas, he appeared triumphantly with them on my tray- procured from first class! Not many people were as astute as one of the nurses at Rosalind's kindergarten, who was instantly sympathetic to her requests on diet, saying that she had had a great deal of trouble when breastfeeding her own daughter (now 17 years old) because she was eating a lot of bran at the time, trouble which only came to an end when she stopped eating bran. Rosalind had the rare pleasure of preaching to the converted.

At this point, fate again took a hand. My third daughter, being a devotee of zinc after it had cured her mouth ulcers, had seen a book called 'The Zinc Solution' by Professor Bryce-Smith of Reading University, and been so impressed she had ordered copies for the entire family. And there, after all the years, was the answer to my riddle, a factor in the bran known as phytic acid.

Memory stirred and turned back thirty years. First to that warning in the Health Department books on mother care. Make sure your child drinks one or more pints of milk a day if he, or she, eats wholemeal flour in any form because of the presence of phytic acid in the bran, which can leach the body of calcium by forming calcium phytate the body cannot absorb. A warning that had since dropped away from baby care books. Second, to the work of Mellanby in 1924 that I had read about when doing my PhD on medical organisation in the 1960's. He had worked on the problem of rickets in Scottish children (a disease with defective utilisation of calcium) and found that the whole grain, oatmeal, caused rickets in his animals far more readily than white flour, or maize.

I read the book avidly. Phytic acid was the chief villain of Professor Bryce-Smith's piece. It not only had the capacity to combine with calcium, as mentioned in the baby care book, but also with other minerals as well- zinc, iron, manganese, magnesium, molybdenum and copper. It made each of them 'biologically

59

unavailable' to the enzyme systems for which they were required, unless there was an excess of any one over the free phytic acid, that could chelate (combine) with them, present at the time.

The mineral which concerned Professor Bryce-Smith most was advertised in the title of the book, namely zinc. This metal has such an extensive role in the function of enzyme systems in the body- at least twenty- any shortage of exogenous zinc must be of serious concern, as protein and starch digestion could both be significantly impaired. Indeed, he argued such a shortage may well be the explanation of a number of still inexplicable disorders.

What is phytic acid, or phytate as it is also called? It is the major part of the phosphorus in the maturing carbohydrate of cereals, legumes (vegetables), pulses (beans), nuts and seeds. It is present in the husk and germ of cereals, but distributed throughout in legumes, pulses, nuts and seeds, including the cereal corn. It is hydrolysed by its own phytase enzymes to inositol and phosphate (important for bone formation), when germination and new growth begins; or by phytase enzymes in the human body.

The first question that rose in my mind as I read Professor Bryce-Smith's book was whether our diet had reduced phytic acid below any level of threat to starch absorption, because it banned all wheat and allied grains unless fermented for six hours. This could be very important to us, because our refined flour diet also meant sacrifice of trace elements and minerals. And there it was, the missing link. The phytic acid level was far higher in commmercial bread made in factories with bread improvers in what was known as the Chorley Wood process than it was in bread made with yeast fermentation over a long period as it had been in cottage bakeries in past generations.

Therefore my family had had an added bonus with their yeast fermented long doughs. These had not only burnt away the maltose, but also reduced the phytic acid as well. Perhaps there was a link between the two, but the only one I noticed as I began to research phytic acid was that rats deficient in zinc developed abnormal glucose tolerance, which disappeared when they had extra zinc. I tested this briefly by taking extra zinc- mindful that the Professor said it was generally deficient in western civilisation, but while my nails grew stronger as evidence of better calcium absorption, my tolerance to maltose was not improved to the point where I could return to normal diet. I wonder what those rats were eating?

A problem of proof of this line of enquiry remained in that phosphorus (and therefore phytic acid) was present in nearly all plants. Many of these were not eaten fermented. I wondered if any other method than fermentation could counteract the ill effects so stringently described by Professor Bryce-Smith?

At this point I went to Ireland in order to have a holiday. While there, I intended to visit Galway University College where a team of doctors and scientists had done major work on aspects of coeliac disease in the Irish, particularly their genetic propensity towards it, one of the highest in the world along with the Swedes and the Austrians.

I had heard about their work quite accidentally. Back in Sydney, I went to a field day on the MacArthur farm at Camden, where I met a biochemist, Dr. Oddy, who was on duty in the building where, in pursuit of alternatives in our family diet as ever, I had made an enquiry as to whether buckwheat was a cereal or not (it is a member of the rhubarb family). By way of explanation, I told him that we responded to coeliac diet, although we were not coeliacs. He remembered papers given by the Galway team at a Dublin conference which he had attended two years before. He gave the reference. I wrote to Professor McNicholl, who sent me back fascinating papers, positing the possibility that the Celts in Ireland, particularly in the north and west, had not evolved as adequate an adaptation to wheat in their diet as the peoples of the Mediterranean borderlands, who had eaten it for nearly four thousand years. My reaction to this thesis was to wonder if people like ourselves, whose ancestry was heavily interlaced with Ireland, could be equally affected. Not by gluten intolerance per se, but by some carbohydrate linkage with the gluten protein, or even by some factor intrinsic to the carbohydrate alone? I conceived the hope that our story might prompt some relevant thought in the coeliac team, despite the fact we clearly had no gluten problem or we could not have eaten the fermented bread.

I was unable to see Professor McNicholl, but a gastro-enterologist, Dr. Stephenson, and a biochemist, Professor Fotrell, were gracious enough to spare me the time. This was particularly generous of Professor Fotrell, as he was currently acting as Vice-Chancellor of the College, and I felt apologetic that the interview proved abortive. I drew a total blank, except for a comment Dr. Stephenson made after Professor Fotrell left. They had patients who appeared to be coeliacs, but who did not entirely respond to the coeliac diet, and they now thought there were several profiles of coeliac disease. But otherwise, the response on their side was an utter blank. My recital dropped into a vacuum. Clearly I was running on an utterly different track.

Never mind, I had made progress in Ireland from quite another source, again by chance. I had dropped in to the Department of Nutrition of the Cork University College to ask if anyone there happened to be researching phytic acid or zinc. Dr. Mulvihill referred me to a Dr. Albert Flynn, who had investigated zinc levels in Irish diet.

Dr. Flynn received me with great courtesy, although I had bounded out of the blue. He was more guarded about the prevalence of zinc deficiency than Professor Bryce Smith- at least in Ireland. But of course, the problems must vary from country to country, according to types of grain, fertilisers used, and natural soil fertility. Dr. Flynn was kind enough to ring me next day. He had remembered a fairly recent article commenting on a Irish National Nutrition Survey to determine why the rate of rickets in children had doubled. This had been carried out for two years during World War 2. He sent me the article. Again, halleluljah! The only difference in the diet of the children studied during the years of the survey was that they had changed from eating white to wholemeal bread. The finding was that phytic acid in the bran was responsible for the calcium deficiency disease, rickets, by combining with the calcium present in the childrens' diet to make it biologically unavailable. It is worthy of note in this context that the scientist Mellanby, already mentioned, and co-workers had only recently identified phytic acid as the 'rachitogenic' (rickets-producing) factor he had nominated as long ago as 1924. It is also worthy of note that not all the children studied were affected. Could the group that were affected be in our category, I wondered, remembering the slight affectation my children had developed in the straight bone formation of their legs? Rosalind, for example, had become quite knock-kneed.

Up to date all my concentration had been on wheat, eaten in British-based diet as bread in greater preponderance than unfermented cakes and biscuits- at least until recent times. Only latterly have families begun to increase the proportion of unfermented wheat with Italian style pastas, spaghettis and pizzas, or breakfast cereals.

But what of similar grains? Rye eaten as bread (often 80% wheat) or biscuits? Barley in soups, and stews, or partly fermented into malt for a dozen uses? Or oatmeal, that staple of Celtic diet for centuries? Oatmeal deserved first consideration, being the one grain still most prominent in western diet as an alternative to wheat, but never fermented.

I started with the conundrum that had struck me when reading the work of the Galway coeliac unit team. Irish people had one of the highest coeliac rates in the world, possibly one in three hundred, because they had not eaten wheat until the time of the potato famine in 1845. But they had eaten the very similar grain, oatmeal, with the same protein, gluten, for hundreds of years. Was there some process they had used to make oatmeal more digestible, the equivalent of fermenting the wheat in Europe, burning and baking the corn, and treating it with the alkaline lime to release the bound niacin (vitamin B3) in Mexico, or baking soda bread with the alkaline bicarbonate of soda for the same purpose as in Ireland? Perhaps they had fermented their oatmeal for several days to make the traditional Scotch dish, 'sowens'. Perhaps they had baked their oatmeal in cobweb thin sheets on a hot griddle like the Scotch oatmeal cakes. Did they use ordinary raw oatmeal when they did?

I had already proved oatmeal was not digestible for us, even with the husk removed. I had obtained a bag of hulled oatmeal fine flour for the experiment with the greatest difficulty. It could only be bought through a wholesaler, as its sole use was in the trade. However, taking delivery of the resultant twenty five kilo bag gave me a chance to talk to an oatmeal chemist, who told me that this hulled oatmeal had only been exposed to steam just long enough to prevent rancidity, which meant that the phytic acid present in it would still be high, irrespective of the inherent maltose. A further problem was that oatmeal had no endogenous phytase enzymes to act on the phytic acid, that is, enzymes contained within itself.

My oldest daughter and I baked the flour into small cakes and pancakes. The result was an unmitigated disaster, the reactions far more severe than I expected. She said the effect lasted for days, affecting her vision, her piles, her temper, her concentration and alertness. I also found very disturbing effects on eyes, hypoglycaemia, and mood.

At this stage, I was quite certain gluten did not affect us. I had undertaken an experiment for a month. This involved combining wheat 'cornflour' starch and gluten to make up a flour which I knew to be free of phytic acid. I had been assured of this by a technician at the plant of Mauri Brothers and Thompson, who

63

said that phytic acid would be spun off in the process that separated starch from gluten, as it was water-soluble. Over a period of six weeks, this combination, consumed daily at breakfast in pancakes, gave me no reactions of any importance. When I had a blood test at Clinical Assays I showed no evidence of gliadin (the toxic fraction of protein to coeliacs) anti-bodies. The next step of course would be to combine cornflour, phytic acid, and gluten, and see what happened. This is a test I have had neither time nor opportunity to make.

I had another inadvertent experiment. While in Ireland, I used an Odlums gluten free flour sold in the supermarkets in making up my recipes. After some weeks, I became increasingly dubious about it, as mild digestive and energy balance problems began to creep up on me. Shades of the Mauri Brothers and Thompson gluten free mix back in Sydney, though this time without the added soya flour.

I rang Odlum's laboratory in Dublin. Was the flour in fact a cornflour, as it seemed to be a coarser grind than cornflour, closer to ordinary plain flour? He could not say. It came from England. He did know it contained some soya flour. If the problem lay in the soya flour, that could bring me back once more to phytic acid, if English, like Australian, soya flour was not thoroughly processed to remove the phytic acid. I was to find out later in Australia that it was not. There were only two or three processing plants in the world that processed soya flour properly, as hexane processing plants are expensive and operate on high demand. However this question did not invalidate the supposition of gradual adverse effects from phytic acid.

I had a brief chance to make a comparison. When I visited Dr. Cummings, a gastroenterologist in the Dunn Nutritional Laboratory in Cambridge, I complained about the Odlums' mix. He gave me a sample of the gluten-free flour they had been using in experiments in their laboratory. It did not have the same ill effect. I have not been able to track down the sources of both flours as yet to compare the milling processes of those flours. If there was no difference, I would only be able to incriminate the soya flour.

In Ireland once more during the summer of 1988, I wrestled again with the vexing problem of oats. We had eaten porridge in the winter in my youth. Had there been something about the way it was prepared that made it more digestible as the long fermentation of our breads had made wheat more digestible? If there was something my mother did, it was in the traditional Irish or British

64

way. She had spent all her early years in London and Ireland. What was the Irish way? I went into the Tourist Bureau at Cork, and began to search through the old Irish cookbooks they sold there as a tourist gimmick (Waterstones had not opened). Not with much hope, as methods of preparation are not usually incorporated in recipe books, but simply handed on in practice. But there it was. The second missing key. There in a traditional Irish recipe for oat flummery often eaten with beer. The oats were steeped for twenty four hours, and the liquid drained off three times. Meanwhile no doubt the mixture was kept at the back of the round-the-clock kitchen fire at a temperature favourable for the breakdown of the starch.

I began to ask the locals. The elderly postmistress at Tower near Blarney said the preparation of oats used to take a long time in the old days. Another Irish lady told me her mother used to soak oats all day, cook them at night, cool them, then reheat them for breakfast next day. Another friend could remember his grandmother doing the same. Yet another said her mother would throw the oats away if they had not been steeped long enough. A Welsh lady told me a different variation. She used to soak oatmeal a long time, then cook them slowly all night on a low fire. Indeed everywhere I asked the story was the same- memory of practices that would be lost a generation later. They seemed a very far cry from present preference for instant, or almost raw, oats. I would dearly have loved to have met Mellanby and asked him in what form he fed oats to his dogs- raw or cooked, or steeped and cooked.

The more I thought about it, the more positively I concluded our grandmothers were not going to all that trouble merely for the love of trouble. They were only following centuries of accumulated wisdom, which is what I now call folk wisdom. How had they acquired that wisdom? By being down on the farm. Animal models served well for humans.

There were two possible reasons for the need for such wisdom. The first that somehow the gluten or protein was modified in the process, which seemed unlikely; the second that the effect of anti-nutrients was modified, chief of which was phytic acid, not so much by their water solubility, as the water is absorbed rather than poured off, but by their sensitivity to heat.

I remembered my mother had always soaked oatmeal, and cooked it for a long time. She had also soaked a number of other foods before cooking them- not only grains and pulses such as barley, lentils, beans and rice, but also tubers like potatoes, parsnips, turnips and so on. Somewhere along the line I had abandoned her custom along with everyone else of my post World War 2 generation. I pondered why. We did so not only for reasons of convenience, but also because we believed our ancestors had cooked the good out of vegetables. We had heeded the nutrionists who said that boiling and prolonged overcooking reduced the vitamins and minerals in food. We had switched to lightly cooked, even raw food, to avoid 'losing the good' as my mother had. I had not imagined for a moment that I was losing some of her wisdom in the process as well, the necessity to counteract some of the bad effects of raw foods as well.

I took myself off to the Library of Cork University College to re-read Mellanby's work. I was suddenly aware he was advancing a powerful argument to force drastic reappraisal of the whole vitamin-mineral argument for whole food, or lightly cooked even raw, food. He argued that the existence of these vitamins and minerals in the raw food did not mean they were necessarily available. He warned a greater deficiency of zinc, calcium, iron, and even phosphorus itself, could be brought about by diets which actually contained more of these substances, so that any analysis of mineral intake could be quite misleading as to the efficacy of the diet in adequately supplying those substances to the tissues. I soon found out that other scientists over the years had endorsed his findings.

The technical details of such discussions are highly specialised, even daunting, but some of the conclusions are not difficult to understand.

1. The anti-nutrient effect of phytic acid in the phosphorus of plant foods means that diets rich in phosphorus are actually deficient in diet phosphorus.
2. The anti-nutrient effect of phytic acid in phosphorus in individual foods can be diminished by dissolving in water, exposing to heat at a low temperature to activate its inherent enzyme, phytase, or heating to a high temperature.
3. The anti-nutrient level of phytic acid in diet as a whole can be reduced by choosing foods with less phosphorus in preference to those with more e.g. white flour or rice instead of wholemeal flour and brown rice. Bananas (with none) instead of other fruits. Root vegetables instead of lentils, and so on.
4. The anti-nutrient effect can be lessened by eating a balanced meal, as by eating eggs, cheese or meat with breakfast cereals,

rather than eating them alone.

As knowledge of anti-nutrients in raw plant foodstuffs grew in the sixties and seventies, many studies came to light showing that the very methods used to reduce them were those elaborated so long ago by our ancestors (some are summarised in Appendix A). They were fermentation, steeping at fireside temperatures, baking at high temperatures, and lengthy cooking or boiling often with added vinegar, wine, salt or bicarbonate of soda. A great deal of cooked food was recycled, such as cold potato, pumpkin, rice, cabbage and so on.

This growing body of evidence by biochemists seemed to indicate that far from bran (fibre) being valuable in our diet, as so enthusiastically claimed on all sides, the reverse may be the case. In fact the very processing of wheat, which causes the loss of nutrients so strongly condemned by health experts, may in fact enhance the biological value of the residual flour, which can, in any case, be fortified to restore some of its original nutritional value as is done in America.

Some researchers challenged any such finding, saying that adaptation to phytic acid is universal, and sufficiently strong to negate the effect of high phytic acid intake. One even proved to his satisfaction there is no effect. Other studies appeared implicating the lignin in bran rather than the phytic acid.

Back to the library with a question that emerged from my conclusion about the folk wisdom of my ancestors. Was raw food basically hostile to man? The title of a book, that cropped up in bibliographies to articles on phytic acid, had first suggested this to me. The title was 'Toxic Constituents of Foodstuffs'. The very sound of the title was ominous, so much so that I deferred reading it until I was certain I had understood what phytic acid was all about. Otherwise I risked making confusion worse confounded. When I did open the book, I was horrified. Phytic acid was only one of several anti-nutrients in food that could interfere with metabolism as phytic acid did.

ANTI-NUTRIENTS

The book, 'The Toxic Constituents of Foodstuffs' is a collection of papers by experts on different aspects of the subject, edited by Irvin Liener. Its message is best summarised by a short assertion made in Cereal Chemistry by Davis (58.5 pp. 454-60). 'Legumes contain such anti-nutritional, or toxic factors as protein inhibitors, phytic acid, tannins and lectins, all of which have the potential to affect protein availability, or be toxic.' An assertion equally applicable to pulses, seeds and leaf foods like tea.

In Liener's introduction to the book, he gives a definition of toxic as meaning a cumulative toxicity that is not so easily identified as the severe poisoning the general public imagines by the word, as with certain species of fish or plants, or invasive bacteria like salmonella or listeria. He elaborates as follows-

'For reasons which scientists have yet to fathom, Nature has seen fit to endow many plants with the capacity to synthesise a wide variety of chemical substances, which are known to exert a deleterious effect when ingested by man or animals.

'It did not require much experience for primitive man to learn to avoid the consumption of those plants, which produced an immediate, unpleasant reaction, and which may even have proved fatal. What could not have been realised by early man, and even today may not be fully appreciated, is the fact that, although there might not be an immediate violent reaction to a certain food, there might still be a slow, cumulative effect resulting in frank disease, or less than optimum health. It is this aspect of the problem that poses the greatest challenge in the future since knowledge of this nature is accumulated very slowly and with difficulty, particularly as the causative principles remain unidentified.

'Although there are some plants which are known to produce a violent expression of poisoning (Kingsbury 1964), what is more commonly observed are much more subtle effects produced only by prolonged ingestion of a given plant. Such effects might include an inhibition of growth, a decrease in food efficiency, a goiterogenic response, pancreatic hypertrophy, hypoglycaemia, liver damage etc. Other factors which should be taken into consideration include the species of animal, its age, size and sex, its state of health and plane of nutrition, and any stress factors that might be superimposed on these variables.

'In other words, the toxic effects of any of these are not necessarily dramatic, not only if the degree of toxicity is low, but also if the toxic effects are partly destroyed as they are in cooking, or common means of preparation. The molecules may be too small to stimulate the nervous system. They may therefore cause minor symptoms, rather than allergic reactions, and, as a consequence, skin and blood tests will be negative and irrelevant. However, the small molecules could find a final common pathway with true allergic reactions, and a wide range of symptoms. And the toxic effects may be more dramatic, if patterns of food preparation and consumption are dramatically changed, and the normal detoxification mechanisms of the body can no longer cope.'

In the last two sentences, staring me in the face was a validation of my findings to date. First, for the cumulative nature of our maltose intolerance problem, and my hypothesis that excess phytic acid (and possibly other anti-nutrients) could well have compounded that problem. Second, for the fact that the problem was further compounded by changes in kitchen practice, both in preparation and styles of cooking.

The day I had left home and the folk-wisdom based habit of my mother from her early days in England and Ireland was the day I had begun the long decline in my health during those years when I followed current fashions culled from a dozen theories and countries, and, at the heart of them, the idea that the closer to nature, the better. I began a new journey backwards towards my ancestral kitchen. No raw foods. No food that was not well-soaked, well-cooked, and cooked to oven temperatures wherever possible.

It is only fair to say some people have doubted the validity of such assertions as that from Liener quoted above, although quite complex studies have been carried out in a number of countries on plant foods of all kinds. This doubt is due to the fact that experimental results have not always been consistent owing to variation in method, and theories have not always coincided. Yet what if Liener's statements are valid? We might reasonably then conclude that plant foods in their raw state are guilty until proved innocent, in other words basically hostile to man; a fact that would appear to have been familiar to our ancestors for centuries. A fact we have lately forgotten.

What are these anti-nutrients? First and foremost, they are natural substances, intrinsic to the dynamics of the plant. They are not additives in any sense, such as those so many diet faddists and band-wagon health experts love to hate. They are widely distributed in all plants with few exceptions.

There are a number of these anti-nutrients, some little understood as yet. They vary in their combinations in different plants. Individually they may vary in their level in the plant according to the cultivar or type- for example hard compared to soft wheat, or long compared to short grain rice; or the type of crop- dry compared to irrigation rice, or even the climate- warm compared to cold years. What is their physiological effect? They have the potential to interfere with the digestion of man, shunting food by-products into sidings and wrong alleys, as it were, with all the potential for ultimate malnutrition.

Now Davis, cited above, names four main categories of anti-nutrients- phytic acid, protein inhibitors, tannins and lectins.

1. PHYTIC ACID

It impairs protein digestion by interacting with digestive enzymes, forming insoluble complexes less subject to proteolytic attack than the same protein alone at both acidic and alkaline pH. It chelates with zinc, iron, calcium, copper, magnesium and manganese.

a) Zinc is essential for protein synthesis, nucleic acid metabolism, cell growth, normal growth hormone levels, behaviour patterns, and protection from toxic elements such as cadmium or lead.
b) Iron is needed in high amounts for red blood corpuscles.
c) Calcium is required for the activity and maximum stability of alpha-amylase in starch digestion.
d) Copper is necessary for iron metabolism, and cross-linking of the amino acid, lysine.
e) Magnesium and manganese are involved with cartilage, oxidation, glucose utilisation, lactose synthesis, and with the nervous system.

A study of Tankong et al., published in 1981, concluded that reduction of phytic acid in whole grain appeared prudent, because other sources of phytic acid, such as vegetable proteins, were being consumed in increasing amounts (Cereal Chemistry 1981 58 pp. 347-50).

This view was echoed in another report of Harland and Prosky that intake of phytic acid increases as intake of dietary fibre from whole grains, fruits, nuts and vegetables is increased (Cereal Chemistry 1979 58(4) pp. 347-50). One is tempted to reach the same conclusion as Dr. Batten, who is trying to breed a strain of

70

wheat lower in grain total phosphorus (it is higher with input of superphosphate fertiliser). He writes 'I consider the reduction and ultimate elimination of phytate from cereals to be a meritorious aim for nutritional reasons' (Cereal Chemistry 63(5) pp. 384-7).

2. INHIBITORS

They are found throughout the plant world, chiefly in the legumes, and then mostly in the seeds. Several types may exist in one plant. They are thought to protect the plants as they ripen by reason of their ability to depress, or inactivate, a variety of enzymes, as well as the digestive amylases in the saliva and pancreas, in their predators, whether insects or humans. They also inhibit the protease enzymes, which digest proteins in the body, because they can inhibit the release of their own soluble dextrins (starch) until the plant reaches maturity. They are of two types, proteinaceous specific to a particular enzyme, and non-proteinaceous inhibitors of a number of quite different enzymes. Very little is known about them.

a) Trypsin and chymo-trypsin inhibitors

They are widely distributed among the cereal grains, including buckwheat, corn and rice. Several are usually present in one plant as polysaccharides. They suppress enzymic trypsin from the pancreas, and alpha-amylase from the saliva and pancreas. There are more in some varieties of a plant than others, more for example in winter than in spring wheat. They exist in beans of all kinds. Most are water soluble and heat sensitive, but this can vary in cultivars of the same species. Some resist heat. Others do not, e.g. lima compared to field beans. Some species have much less than others, e.g. wholewheat flour compared to raw soybean meal. What does seem true for all species is that the speed of destruction increases as the heat rises, e.g. what takes two hours at 90 degrees can be accomplished in 10 minutes at 120 degrees.

A great deal of work has been carried out on various types of beans, because of their importance as the main source of protein in Africa and Asia. Research on soybeans as early as 1917 showed that heat treatment improved their nutritive value (J. Biol. Chem. 1917 32 pp. 369-387). Rats grew 15%-20% faster, when twelve different varieties of phaseolus beans were autoclaved (steam cooked) to inactivate inhibitors, than when those same beans were untreated (Cereal Chemistry 1973 58 pp. 454-60). Soybeans in the East are habitually well-processed before consumption, tofu in Indonesia for example in four different stages. Soybeans are also

71

extensively processed in America by hexane (alcohol) treatment before feeding to animals and humans (less in some countries).

b) Alpha-amylase inhibitors

They inhibit alpha-amylase enzymes both in the saliva and the pancreas. They are soluble proteins in wheat, particularly hard winterwheat, rye and taro root. They slow down germination of wheat exposed to unseasonable rain or heat, so that plant breeders are trying to breed varieties of wheat with more rather than less inhibitors. They were once thought to be limited, but are now known to be widespread in nature. Maize has little. Sucrose none. But there are large amounts in some cultivars of wheat. Several are active against proteases like trypsin as well as alpha-amylase. They are significant in human nutritional terms, as they decrease starch availability significantly. Some of the starch may then be fermented by intestinal microflora, and absorption of fermentation products (e.g. acetic and butyric acids) would then follow (Enzymes 1987 ed. Kruger et al. p. 185).

They have relative thermal stability, and may persist through baking and cooking. They are found in a considerable number of cooked cereal foodstuffs. 10-20 % of their original activity towards human salivary alpha-amylase has been found in baked wheat and rye bread. On the other hand, less than 2% is present in spaghetti after 15 minutes boiling.(J. Am. Chem. Society 65 p.1247).

c) Invertase inhibitors

They impair sucrose digestion by suppressing the invertase enzymes that split sucrose into fructose and glucose. They exist in a wide variety of plants such as potatoes, beet and corn.

d) Cholinesterase inhibitors

Solanine is found in tubers (carrots, turnips, radish, potatoes and beet), fruit (eggplant, orange, apple), and greens (celery, asparagus, broccoli). It is most highly concentrated in the skin and sprouts, and particularly high in green potatoes, when it can be over ten times as high as in mature potatoes. It is not destroyed by cooking.

e) Glucosides.

(i). Goitrogens

These can be inactivated by heat, or by increasing the iodine content, as shown by studies in rats and poultry. They can also be neutralised by casein (milk) irrespective of any extra iodine.

Rats fed soybean baby food showed an enlargement of the

thyroid where the iodine level was too low (Block et al. Arch Biophys. 1961 93 pp. 15-24).

a) Thio-glucosides

They are potent thyroid inhibitors found in plants of the Cruciferae family, which are common in cattle feed and in human diet- e.g. cabbage, brussels sprouts, broccoli, turnips, cauliflower, and garden cress.

The highest concentration is in the mature seed. They are also in mustard and horse-radish, giving them their distinctive flavour.

Scientists are concerned they may cause endemic goitre through transmission in milk and beef from cattle fed kale.

b) Non-thio-glucosides

These are present in skins of nuts such as peanuts, cashew and almond, and in soybeans.

(ii). Cyanogetic glucosides

These are mainly three types, almost universal among plants. Vitamin B12 may play an active role in its detoxification in the upper gastric tract. They are found in sweet potatoes, yam, maize, millet, sugar cane, peas, beans of all types, bamboo shoots, and the kernels of a number of fruit, (including apple and lemon). Cyanogetic plants should not be stored for long periods.

Cooking practice is important e.g. cassava (tapioca).

(iii). Saponins

They occur in a wide variety of plants. They are in soybeans, beets, spinach, asparagus, alfalfa, yams, peanuts and green tea. They are also in soft drinks, beers, confections, soaps and shampoos. They inhibit certain digestive enzymes and cholinesterase, but this is thought to be counteracted by proteins present. Certainly a study of saponins in soybeans showed they were harmless to chickens and rats at fairly high levels. They hemolyze red cells, and may form complexes with cholesterol which help to reduce liver and serum cholesterol.

3. LECTINS

Not all lectins are toxic, although ten are. The toxic lectins can agglutinate (clump) red cells in human blood. Such lectins are present in certain beans in human diet e.g. the red and black (with the toxic A type lectin) compared to the white beans, lentils and peas (with the non-toxic D type). The same is true of other plants where they are found- seeds, roots, tubers, leaves and potatoes.

They are water soluble and sensitive to heat, particularly to wet heat at autoclaving temperature of 120 degrees and above. However the most toxic are the most heat resistant, and can agglutinate after 45 minutes at such temperatures. These need to be cooked traditionally that is, soaked, the water thrown away, then boiled for a long time.

4. TANNINS

These are as capable of inactivating a series of enzymes, including salivary and pancreatic amylase and trypsin, as alpha amylase inhibitors of wheat and rye. They can also inhibit iron absorption, although this effect can be neutralised by the casein of milk products, or advantaged by ascorbic acid. They are a diverse group of polyphenolic compounds present in many vegetable foods, particularly those with yellow flowers. Information about them is limited.

Examples of food with high tannin content are tea, beans, peas, lentils, sunflower seeds, carob, yellow peas, spinach, wheat germ and aubergine; and with low tannin content, carrots, potatoes, tomatoes.

5. CASEIN INHIBITORS

They exist in several food gums.

6. OTHER SUSPECT FACTORS

a) Citral
This is a constituent of orange oil which can prevent absorption of fat-soluble vitamins, and possibly in excess cause damage to blood vessels, and contribute to cardiovascular disease. It is present in orange skin and therefore found in orange juices flavoured with orange oil, marmalade, or orange drinks from compressed whole fruit. White mineral oil is used in the baking industry as an adjunct to efficient processing and can migrate into the finished product.

b) Salicylates
These are small organic molecules which occur in many fruits and vegetables. They tend to cause pharmacological, rather than allergic reactions. Adverse reactions are dose related, and only occur in sensitive individuals who have a constitutional predisposition. Identification of foods is often difficult.

c) Benzoates
These are similar to salicylates. Among the foods where they are to be found are tea, peppermint, honey, licorice, herbs and spices.

d) Pressor Amines
They are aromatic amino compounds such as serotonin and norepinephrine, which act as potent vasoconstrictors and thereby elevate the blood pressure.
However it appears that the bacterial degradation of these amines in the intestinal tract can easily cope with the amounts consumed in western diet. They are found in chocolate, pineapple juice, avocado, alcohol and cheese.

e) Monosodiumglutamate
There are large variations in the concentration of MSG in fresh or processed food, or even in the same food depending on its age, as for example in the ripening of tomatoes. It is very high in stock cubes, crisps, tomato paste, and blue vein, cheddar or camembert cheese.

f) Pectins
They are potent in apples and lemons, particularly the latter.

g) Raffinose and Stachyose
They are oligosaccharides, which are fermented by microbial action in the colon, producing gases and hence flatus. For this reason, they have been said to have been the cause of side-effects from industrial glucose syrup noted in some individuals. They are present in beans, whose ability to cause flatus is well-documented. They exist in wheat and oat bran, but the amount is much greater in wheat bran. The amount in sweet potato is greater than other legumes. They diminish as the plant grows, and almost completely disappeared by maturity.

By the time I had finished reading 'Toxic Constituents of Foodstuffs', I had a complete rationale for swearing off raw salads forever, let alone those raw carrot sticks and cauliflower florets I am so often offered at cocktail parties nowadays. I had always hated salads. They had never appeared on my mother's table in my youth, and I thankfully banished them from mine except for the odd occasion.

Of course, in the past I had dutifully eaten raw or lightly cooked foods on the popular presumption that primitive peoples had always lived close to nature, and so should we. Was this really true? Having questioned all other sacred cows, it was time to question this one as well.

I began with my own area. I found that Australian aborigines, Melanesians, and Polynesians alike rarely ate food raw, and not only cooked vegetables at higher temperatures than boiling by steaming or baking in earth ovens, but also often prepared them at some length, as with coconuts and yams. Some of the foods they ate raw, such as bananas, had a very low phytic acid level, or none.

Asians seldom eat raw vegetables or brown rice. Vegetables are usually cooked well, or in the highly focussed heat of a wok. Rice is soaked, the water thrown away, then boiled, baked or fried. The husks or bran are fed to the pigs. Brown rice, they say, is indigestible. Soya beans are cooked in many ways, and often either cultured or fermented.

Indians often cook foods for a lengthy time. Greeks soak and boil beans for some hours. West Africans process corn for days. Taiwanese farmers boil sweet potatoes before giving them to pigs as food. American Hopi Indians picked corn green and dried it to make bound niacin available. The list is endless. The conclusion is obvious. Raw food was generally treated with the utmost caution in traditional societies.

I came across curious idiosyncracies of national diet that invited explanation. For example, the use of coconut milk to cook vegetables in New Guinea and Fiji, or the use of vinegar in cooking in Central European cultures. The significance, if any, of yoghurt in Indian and Bulgarian cookery. The common use of cream buttermilk in Irish cuisine. I resisted the allure of these riddles. While I would have loved to travel the world collecting cooking folk-lore, the answer to the biochemical validity of these practices with raw foods lay in books and journals.

I now had a simple truth that could easily be unravelled in those books, and a truth that could readily be explained to ordinary uncomplicated people around me, who knew nothing about the complicated world of science, and got a dazed look on their faces at the mere sound of words like phytic acid- a reaction my daughters assure me they shared. Our bodies were our inheritance from our ancestors. Those bodies had been adapted to the way of life they had evolved. If we moved away from that way of life, and abandoned the diet of our ancestors, we did so at our own risk. The only road to good health was the road laid down long ago.

By this time I was driven inescapably to the conclusion most of the problems my family had suffered had arisen from a reckless and thoughtless abandonment of the customs and the diet of my ancestors. They had learnt to beware of all plant life in its native state as inherently indigestible. They had come by the wisdom evident in the domestic practice of their cooking, and the balances of their diet, through trial and error over many centuries. They soaked all their vegetables and most grains. They baked a good deal of their food. They steamed puddings and custards. They ate compound meals wherever possible including breakfast (starch with fat and protein). They ate a wider variety of starches, with arrowroot, sago, tapioca and ground rice. They consumed only limited quantities of fruit and fruitjuice. They made their own sweets. They fermented and baked their own bread in a leisurely process.

I can see my mother's kitchen still with her great kitchen table. The toffees and the coconut ice for birthday parties. The bottling of fruit from the orchard, and home made lemonade or ginger beer. The constant repertoire of biscuits, scones and cakes. The frequent sponges. The blancmanges and the apple sagos. And on and on. The ancient village tradition of cooking we have lost, and with it health and common sense and all the camaraderie of a growing up household. All replaced by a supermarket without a heart.

However, there was a worm even at the centre of this apple. My mother's diet undoubtedly was much better for myself and my family in that it minimised the potential effect of anti-nutrients and other possible antagonists to efficient carbohydrate metabolism- as it had in my youth. But we lived in a world where we could not isolate ourselves from what was in other people's kitchens. The children daily ran a gauntlet of food loaded with that creeping invasion of glucose (maltose) syrup, or occasionally merely glucose, which so readily upset the delicate balance of their glucose metabolism.

To contain that balance, we had to have working rules, some of which were similar to those classified by nutritionists as suitable for people with 'impaired glucose tolerance', and others not.

'SUGARS'

I have already mentioned my blind trials with sucrose, maltose, fructose, galactose and glucose, the first two of which are disaccharides, and the last three of which are monosaccharides. I recorded effects from maltose, galactose and glucose, but none from sucrose or fructose. It is timely to discuss all of these. I will deal first with the sugars I found 'benign', namely sucrose and fructose.

When I first realised sucrose was acceptable in our diet, as long as the fraction of inverted sugar- half glucose, half fructose- was kept fairly low, I was surprised. Being anti-sucrose was then all the rage, with the campaign to reduce dental caries. Professor Yudkin's books, which blamed sucrose for much evil were highly regarded. I already knew from the tests done on the children in Melbourne that they had no identifiable reaction to fructose. I also knew that fructose was said to be more acceptable to diabetics than sucrose.

Therefore it was something of a surprise to read the comments of Professor Truswell of the Department of Nutrition of the University of Sydney which confirmed my own once unfashionable view. Sucrose, he said, had a better claim to be called a natural food than many other foods, since it was free from mutagens, carcinogens, pathogens and mycotoxins. He pointed out that its constituent monosaccharides, fructose and glucose, are the main intravenous foods, and effective in oral rehydration; and that neoborn infants preferred sucrose over glucose solution at birth.

Indeed, sucrose no longer seemed to be the villain it had once been. In 1979, the American Clinical Society of Nutrition had a task force of nine experienced researchers examine the evidence on six dietary factors that were thought to bear heavily on a number of major degenerative changes. Of the ten sets of votes they took, carbohydrate and sucrose scored lowest, a mean 11 out of 100. In 1987, a circular sent to two hundred experts named sucrose as only sixth of possible causes of diabetes, blood pressure, and heart disease.

In reporting this, Professor Truswell pointed out it was easier to make rats fat with high fat diets than high sugar diets; while diabetes was highest in countries with low carbohydrate but high fat intake. (Food and Tech. in Aust. 1987 39 pp. 134-42). There was no plausible mechanism from animal experiments whereby sucrose could lead to coronary heart disease.

79

This finding, if correct, is of enormous importance in view of the wholesale replacement of sucrose by glucose syrup in processed supermarket foods in recent times; substituting a substance we had found highly inimical for one we had found relatively benign. The odd disturbing report, adverse to glucose syrup, vanished into oblivion. For example, that animals given 10% glucose in water gained more weight than those given water. Or that mild degrees of hypoglycaemia, or nausea and dizziness, even vomiting in glucose tolerance tests were by no means uncommon. I myself had had a severe migraine, vomiting, and disorientation in my test in 1988.

No attempt had been made to relate any reports to glucose syrup, partly because glucose syrup contains a very large number of component sugars, and partly because workers in the industry have tended to attribute any ill effect to the presence of certain rare food sugars, like raffinose and stachyose, which are capable of causing flatus. They are thought to be in such minute quantities as to cause no danger despite their extreme toxicity.

Glucose syrup had come to be preferred in baby formulae on the basis that it was less threatening to teeth than sucrose; and in other foods on the basis it was not threatening at all. This fact would be alarming in itself if glucose syrup consisted entirely of the monosaccharide, glucose, but despite its name, it is not. In fact, glucose syrup is glucose plus fractions of malto/dextrins or disaccharides.

The more one delves into the subject of glucose syrup, the more complicated it becomes. There is not simply one glucose syrup, but a whole range of glucose syrups with different fractions of malto-dextrins according to their end use. If I had not been the victim of the food technology engineering that produces this range, I would have been open-mouthed with admiration that science could work out how to create such a variety of mixtures out of the same basic substance- corn or wheat starch, but not sugar- capable of quite different applications. All with consumer benefit in mind- to prevent adverse effects such as melting in icecream, stickiness and mottling in sweets, breaking in biscuits; to perfect texture and create bulk in products like Aktavite and Ovaltine; to create clearer glazes in desserts; and to ensure viscosity, bulk and economy of price with ice-cream.

The composition of the different glucose syrups is identified by a denominator known as the Dextrose Equivalent. This has a scale 10-70, which is the expression of the sweetness, or viscosity, of a purified aqueous solution of nutritive saccharides of DE20 or more obtained by the hydrolysis of the original starch, rather than the relative concentration of monosaccharides and disaccharides. Viscosity decreases, and solubility increases significantly with increasing DE. At one end of the scale are malto-dextrins with a DE equivalent of less than 20. At the other end is dextrose, syrup or spray dried, with a DE of 100. To complicate matters further, the saccharide composition of productions with the same DE may vary greatly depending on the conditions of hydrolysis. Maltose is the main ingredient in the range of DE 43-52, with 30-59% maltose, and 4-10% glucose. Glucose syrup can be 20% glucose, 63% dextrins, and 17% maltose.

Therefore it can be seen that the term Dextrose Equivalent bears no relation to the actual dextrose content, but is highly technical. It is purely related to the total reducing power of all 'sugars' present towards Fehlings solution. The broad headings used in labelling food products, namely malto-dextrins, glucose, and glucose syrup, cover a wider complexity than would appear; a variety I have had to combine under the one heading as 'glucose syrups' for convenience of argument.

On the basis of the belief that none of these glucose syrups are harmful in any way, they are now used extensively in every product as a quick tour of any supermarket shelves will show. This means that the daily load of intake of glucose and malto-dextrins is astronomically higher than it was two generations ago. I have no doubt that the myriad shoppers that read any one of the descriptions 'glucose' or 'glucose syrup' everywhere on the labels would think blithely that this was a substance with harmless connotations, as in preparations for athletes and invalids. And they would pass over any label that said 'malto-dextrins' as lightly, because the word 'malt' carries an ancient reputation as benefiting health, while the word 'dextrins' is suggestive of dextrose. And I cannot, in all fairness, launch any tirade against food technologists for this. Let it be said, in favour of manufacturers, that they offer glucose syrup in all good faith that all they have done is manipulate a perfectly natural substance. And who is complaining? Only one small voice, mine.

I am convinced very few people really understand what the word 'glucose' really stands for. Glucose is a monosaccharide, a simple molecule, the end product of the breakdown of starch in the original plantfoods. There is very little free glucose in nature. Most occurs in very ripe fruit, grapes, wine and honey. There are insignificant amounts elsewhere. Therefore, normally the body must break starch down to glucose by the action of amylase enzymes from the saliva and pancreas. The subsequent glucose is then actively absorbed by cells in membrane lining the upper small intestine, and transported rapidly into the bloodstream to maintain the necessary levels for the metabolism to function properly. Insulin, released from the pancreas, polices the level to prevent this concentration of glucose in the blood rising too high, removing any excess to store it as glycogen in the 'bank' of the liver. The level of the rise depends on the foods that have been eaten, though in this context it should be noted that fructose, compared to other sugars, does not require insulin release to move through the membrane of the small intestine, but is passively moved by diffusion.

The speed of intake of glucose and the subsequent rise in the blood is, of course, a subject of serious concern for diabetics, who have suffered a 'burn-out' of the capacity of their pancreas to manufacture insulin. It is also important to those classified as non-insulin dependent diabetics, who have merely to monitor their diet carefully; and for those nominated as having impaired glucose tolerance from various causes such as operations. It could equally be important to myself, and my family, who had exhibited the hypoglycaemia of the 'pre-diabetic' as I called it, with loads of glucose syrup, and had diabetes lurking in their ancestral history.

I sidetracked to explore the research done on the subject of metabolic response to ingested carbohydrates (simple and complex) for any light on our problems. I found there was still much disagreement over the effect of simple and complex meals; still much to learn of digestion, transit time, and endocrine response (Jenkins et al. Diabetic Care 1988 112 p. 156). Indeed, debate had become less clearcut than it had been in earlier years, when it was believed that all complex starches were digested similarly, and more slowly, than simple sugars like sucrose. This had been found to be untrue, as numerous comparative studies were made. One for example found that the speed of digestive response for sucrose could be lower than for a wide range of other carbohydrates, such as cooked potato, bread or cornflakes.

In order to establish a consistent basis for research, a 'glycaemic index' was developed, which is the amount of insulin needed to clear an equivalent amount of plasma glucose. This produced interesting results.

1. Breakfast cereals, wheat, oats, rice, and potato rated over 50.
2. Rye, bread, spaghetti, pasta, wholemeal grains, and fruit over 40.
3. Some vegetables, legumes, and dairy products under 40.

Added salt in commercial canning raised the index 10%, while added fat reduced it. Phytic acid reacted negatively. (Behall et al. Am. J. Clin. Nutrition 1988 41 pp. 428-32).

These results were clearly not consistent with our experience, which would have led me to draw up a somewhat different hypoglycaemic chart, one that had more in common with another experiment whereby the glucose/insulin response of 26 subjects was studied to fructose, glucose and sucrose. Ten of these were normal, ten were non-insulin dependent diabetics, and six had impaired glucose tolerance. The response from the three in descending order was glucose, sucrose, fructose; while the response from all three was lower in a complex product than it was from ice-cream or from cake. A puzzling feature of this experiment was that the difference between the contents of the ice-cream and the cake was not large enough to account for the difference in the glycaemic response.

I was intrigued to come across an article on this subject by Dr. Brand at a special symposium in conjunction with the 37th Annual Conference of the Cereal Chemistry Division of the Royal Australian Chemical Institute in 1987, which gave a table listing 'sugars' in terms of their glycaemic response, in which maltose rated highest, lactose next- both of which were the sugars that had to be reduced in our diet- with glucose and sucrose lower in the scale. Exactly in conformity with our practical experience. Yet I saw little pursuit of any line of enquiry on maltose in journals anywhere, hunt though I may. And diets designed to lower glycaemic response were actually diets that could enhance the maltose levels in my book.

I became fascinated by yet another aspect of the subject. Starch high in amylose was said to be digested more slowly , and at a more even rate, than starch high in amylopectin. Should we therefore choose high amylose foods- whatever that might mean- rather than the latter? If so, how did such a list compare with the glycaemic index list? Not all of the foods with little or no amylose were on the high glycaemic list e.g. oats, millet and lentils. Not all of the foods high in amylose were on the low glycaemic list e.g. potato, and rice. In the current state of research, it threw no light on my problems.

Before leaving the subject, I should define the terms amylose and amylopectin. They denote the linear and branched polysaccharides of starch, the former being straight, and the latter being with branching junctions. The branching junctions were once thought to slow down digestion. But evidence now shows that digestion is slower, and the glucose response flatter, when the amylose starch is the highest fraction.

Nearly all starches contain both amylose and amylopectin, but the percentage of each can vary widely between different species and the cultivars of the same species. But in general all non-mutant starches have less amylose than amylopectin, the amylose from a range of species varying between 11% to 37%, or even higher depending on age, season, and weather.

Quite accidentally I found a third factor in slowing down the rate of digestion That was resistant starch. The moment I heard about it I recognised its consistency with what worked for us.

I had called rather tentatively to see Dr. J. Cummings at the Dunn Nutritional Institute in Cambridge with an introduction from Professor Fraser. Dr. Cummings was generous enough to give me a couple of hours of his valuable time in the summer of 1988. I was full of enthusiasm for my ideas on the undesirable effect of anti-nutrients in interfering with starch digestion. My focus was on phytic acid in particular, as the arch-villain of the rest, with the qualification that whatever was effective against one tended to be effective against most.

I did not immediately see the relevance of Dr. Cummings' conjoint work with Dr. Englyst on retrograde starch in the articles he handed me until I returned to London, and had a chance to read them. I was still elated over the significance of his parting words, 'Phytic acid could be an allergen', although I still did not fully understand the relevance until I returned home and Professor Fraser explained it to me. More of that later.

But the work of these two research scientists seems immensely important to me. Their definition of retrograde starch was that percentage of the starch gelatinised in cooking which had become resistant to hydrolysis by alpha-amylase in the small intestine, and passed on to be digested in the large intestine, where it had a fibre effect. The proportion of resistant starch was by no means small. It actually rose higher than non-resistant starch several-fold in many meals they tested (Am. J. Clin. Nutrition 45 pp. 1243-55).

84

Resistant starch could, it seemed, be created by industrial food processing (freezing, freeze drying), or domestic preparation (slow or long cooking, or by reheating (e.g. potatoes, oatmeal, cabbage, even bread), or by choice of suitable foods (bananas for crystalline structure). This theory gave the first reasonable explanation I had seen as to why our ancestors had had no cause to munch their way through muesli and brans to gain a fibre component in their diet. They were effectively gaining a fibre effect from resources other than that part of food normally classified as fibre, such as the husks of grains, by traditional cooking. 'Folk' cooking had a much higher quota of recycled food, or slowly cooked food.

Needless to say, these findings came as an enormous relief to me. Here I had been despised for years for rejecting whole grains and muesli, and eating white everything, when all the time I had been doing just as well with my rehashed potato in potato cakes, my reheated casseroles, and many other traditional foods. Where do you get your fibre, my fibre-mad friends would say? There's just as much in cauliflower, or potato I would say. Or sometimes in exasperation I might protest there was no food value in fibre per se, only roughage, and that in my opinion it probably was a vicious cycle to cure symptoms it produced in the first place. I was only able to add other arguments to the opposition debate in recent months like indigestible lignin binding bile and acid salts, or anti-nutrients.

Dr. Cummings had resolved yet another paradox for me, the reason why potatoes gave us no symptoms, although they rated so high on the glycaemic index. The usual methods of cooking were such as to gelatinise and therefore to retrograde the starch. Once again it was a question of thorough cooking to ensure that result, as in my mother's day. Once again the dynamics of the food were all-important. Potatoes could not be condemned out of hand because they rated high on the glycaemic index. One must ask the question under what conditions were those potatoes tested? Were they chips or boiled potatoes? Were they cooked for a short or long time?

However, while I had unqualified enthusiasm for Dr. Cummings' research, he had a more qualified judgement of my observations. When Professor Fraser checked with him as to whether he had in fact said phytic acid could be an allergen, he had said this was so, but he could not accept my account of the adverse effect of glucose. Oh well! That was nothing new to me, and did not diminish my respect for him. I could understand the reservations of a man of his stature. I had no laboratory proof.

Professor Fraser explained the point of the phytic acid question to me. It was that phytic acid is a small molecule not usually thought to be likely to intrude as an allergen. However, it was thought that small molecules could piggyback on large molecules in the first instance, and thereafter become allergenic in their own right. Whether this were relevant to anything I had observed was, of course, beyond my technical understanding. I could only rest on the fact that, in our case, anti-nutrients and maltose had a bearing on each other; and traditional home cooking gave a satisfactory resolution without hypoglycaemia.

Whereas any expert would still take the view that our maltose problem is a rare problem, this would not be the case with our very much milder lactose problem. Suffice to say here, that I had a specific reaction to galactose (the product of the inversion of lactose along with glucose) in my blind trial with Professor Fraser, and my second grandson in a brief trial with lactose reduced milk; and that lactose intolerance is quite high even in western societies. It is said to be as high as some thirty per cent in Britain. As any remarks I may make on our lactose intolerance have a much wider application, it is worth sparing a little space for the subject.

LACTOSE INTOLERANCE

Anyone reading this account may think I am being excessive in claiming lactose intolerance as well as maltose intolerance. In fact, I thought I was being excessive at first as I was forced from one restriction to another, first wheat and allied grains, then glucose syrup, glucose, and finally after all that, to milk in its various guises.

The no-wheat diet had meant leaving out all items on the coeliac list. The low glucose syrup and glucose diet meant leaving out more than half the ready-made foods still allowed on the coeliac list. The low-milk diet meant all but excluding milk.

I had had only modified that list in two respects. The first by introducing 'long-dough' wheat bread. I have already explained the rationale for this. The second by reducing milk, not removing it altogether. The retention of some milk in the diet was possible for all the family, except in the case of the infancy of my fourth daughter when she became so ill a switch to soymilk formula became imperative.

I was obliged to review my policy on milk with the irruption of seven grandchildren into my life. Problems arose with milk formulae when they were babies. I felt I could not wholly attribute these problems to a shift in infant formulae from sucrose to glucose syrup, malto-dextrins or corn syrup (glucose syrup), as it was variously labelled on food tins and packets. I believed the problems were also partly due to an intolerance to some aspect of milk I had not yet identified. By this time I had rejected the theory that had once been fashionable, that allergy was due to the casein of the milk which differed significantly from human milk. This theory scarcely seemed to fit the fact that milk in one formula was acceptable and not in others, or that the children exhibited a degree of variation in their tolerance, depending on the glucose syrup content of the formula.

They certainly tolerated milk well enough, although they did not digest it as comfortably as other children. They had more frequent motions, and were more restless at night, or in their daytime behaviour, than they ought to have been without milk. However the nutritional value of milk could not be lightly set aside, and the fact the balance of nutrition was much more difficult to achieve in other ways by the amateurism of a mother.

When the grandchildren began to arrive, the same cycle of patchy milk tolerance exhibited by their mothers began to repeat itself. But there were some baffling aspects to their milk intolerance, which I had not noticed with their mothers a generation earlier; as for instance with Emily (now 8) and Alexander (now 4).

Emily's asthma became established after she was five. At that age we had all but banished the asthma by reducing the maltose factor to an absolute minimum, but the final perfection of the diet only came by major limitation of milk (at age 7). Cheese and butter were tolerated better. Alexander had not tolerated any milk formula well, whether with sucrose replacement for corn syrup or not, although it contained added whey (more of this later). He had however tolerated a goat's milk formula. When Alexander was 3, his mother realised that a glass of milk by itself could cause behaviour disorder suggestive of a failure to metabolise it properly.

His cousin Rebecca (now aged 5) had been on soymilk formula, but had migrated to an average intake of milk and cheese after she grew out of the bottle, as my youngest daughter had.

Young Mark survived on the Wyeth formula of S26. Everything else was disastrous, including goat's milk. By the time he was two his mother was scaling down his milk to the lowest possible point, as he began to take solids well. He had always been wakeful at night, and restless by day. But she had felt it was such an excellent source of balanced protein, vitamins and minerals, she had been reluctant to withdraw this most basic infant resource.

As I tried to find a common denominator in the profiles of the various children, I had no clear moment of revelation as I had twice had in solving the problem of maltose intolerance. I had at first no specific answer to my childrens' questions- what could their children have or not have to eat?

By observation I was sure of only two points.
a) The level of tolerance varied in any one of the children, or myself.
b) The level of tolerance depended on how and when the milk was consumed.
   i. by itself.
   ii. if cooked in a high starch pudding (e.g. rice pudding).
   iii. if skimmed, condensed, powdered.
c) the level of tolerance seemed to be lower after the age of 2 or 3.

And I had, by this time, found I reacted to five grammes of galactose in the blind trial I had done for Professor Fraser. Since galactose is the monosaccharide split in the inversion of lactose along with glucose, (further converted into glucose also in the liver), this finding had switched suspicion from casein to lactose, otherwise known as the sugar of milk. Lactose intolerance was a much more likely thesis in view of our susceptibility to the disaccharide, maltose. Was this quite a separate problem, or was there a link between the two as I had always vaguely suspected? This problem was left until last.

When at last I found an entire book on lactose intolerance, I was as astonished as I had been by the book 'Toxic Constituents of Foodstuffs' (ed. Liener). This book was 'Lactose Digestion' (ed. Paige and Bayliss). It comprised a series of papers on the clinical and nutritional implications of lactose intolerance issued by the John Hopkins University Press in 1981. These papers were the fruit of what Dr. Stephenson said was a decade that had been 'an exciting and fruitful one in the area of lactose research' (p. 141).

First as to the prevalence of lactose intolerance. This is extremely high in all traditional zones of non-milking, and even in Europe, the continent of dairying, the prevalence was rated as high as 11% on average. But even higher figures were given for England (20-30%) and France (40%) compared to Negroes (73%).

Second, as to whether the lactase enzymes necessary to convert lactose are constant, the answer is no. The capacity of many people declines from the ages 3 to 5, and even more in adulthood.

Third, as to whether intolerance itself is a constant for milk, no matter how it is consumed, the anwer is no. Intolerance depends on the form in which the milk appears in the diet.
a) Whole milk is better than skim.
b) Milk with a meal is better than milk without a meal.
 c) Milk when turned into buttermilk, yoghurt, or cheese is acceptable depending on the type.
d) Milk when consumed in small quantities through the day, as in tea, is better than when drained at once, even in a person who will produce symptoms after one cup of milk.
e) Milk can be tolerable but not whey, which is a crude solution of lactose.

Fourth, as to whether ingestion of lactose can result in a lower blood glucose response than normal with other foods? The answer is yes.

Fifth, do the lactose levels vary according to the form of milk or milk products? The answer is yes.

For these reasons, the authors in the book are extremely guarded about removing all milk, and milk products, from the diet. They agree that casual elimination could lead to nutritional deficiency. They emphasise that-

a) The amount of lactose needed to provoke symptoms is still in dispute.

b) Milk is an excellent compact source of nutriment.

c) There is not enough information about the balance of nutrients in alternatives.

d) Milk can be selectively consumed according to the amount of lactose present.

e) 'Many people have concluded erroneously that lactose intolerance is synonymous with milk intolerance. It is imperative that these terms should not be used interchangeably' (Dr. Alpers op cit. p. 265).

Most important to myself and my family, who had always seen our problem as one of carbohydrate dynamics, was a highly technical discussion of a number of factors which could affect lactose absorption in the body by acting on the lactase enzyme. It stated that hydrolytic digestion of other disaccharides, eaten at a meal containing lactose, could inhibit lactose hydrolysis by lactase enzymes.

According to Dr. Alpers, 'sucrose or maltose are hydrolyzed into their component sugars, and those component sugars can inhibit further lactose hydrolysis. Thus, lactose hydrolysis is affected not only by the monosaccharides ingested, and by the monosaccharides derived from lactose, but also by the monosaccharides derived from other carbohydrates (sucrose and maltose)... Inhibition of lactase activity may be a factor in producing some of the variable results of standard lactose tolerance tests, and in affecting tolerance to different doses of lactose. Moreover it may play a role in the alteration of lactose intolerance noted when milk is ingested with other foods' (pp. 59-61).

The conclusion was clear enough, although the evidence was highly technical. It asserted the interbalance of these disaccharides, which are so often presented together in composite foods, thus confirming my instinctive reaction so many years earlier. It was possible to develop a scale of choices of icecream according to the type of glucose syrup used. We found Streets icecream, which then contained a lower conversion glucose syrup (lower maltose level), better than Peters with its much higher conversion glucose syrup (higher maltose level), and Dairy Farmers best of all with its no glucose syrup. (This changed when the company was bought out by Peters, when glucose syrup was added). I also attempted to balance off components when faced with normal food when away from home. However, in those early days, I had been extremely vague about any distinctions there might be about the milk content.

I now found out there were decided differences between various milk products, as for example between various ice-creams or yoghurts. Some used more cream than others. Some used added milk powder. Some used extra skimmed milk powder. The same was true for yoghurts, buttermilks, and even cheeses. I was now about to learn a great deal of difference could exist in lactose levels in any given product, depending on the ingredient used- but not from the book on lactose digestion. I had to turn to books on the technology of milk processing. I found such books quite fascinating in that they solved so many riddles that had existed in our observation about milk.

Lactose is normally 40% of the total solids in milk, and does not vary as between the milk of sheep, cows or goats. But this percentage rises to more than half in the residues from cream, cheese, or butter-making such as skimmed milk, whey or buttermilk, unless the buttermilk is a cream buttermilk as was often used in Irish cooking of yore. It is lower in whole milk and even lower in cream, whether sweet or sour, or yoghurt in which the lactose is decomposed by bacteria into lactic acid. It is almost non-existent in butter or cheese.

Commercial buttermilk is usually made from the fermentation of skimmed milk, and this fermentation effectively reduces the lactose level of the skimmed milk some 10-15%. However this figure would change if dried or condensed milk were added, as is often the case. Then the lactose level would again be higher. The same is true of yoghurt, as evaporated whole milk, or dried milk, are often added. Plainly, it is impossible to guess at lactose levels of any such products unless one knows what combination of types of milk have been used in their manufacture. It is best to avoid them. Certainly my second daughter, Leone, has an extremely low tolerance to dried milk in products like coffee and tea whiteners.

Lactose levels are still a minefield for the lactose intolerant as can be seen from the following table.

Milk-

Plain condensed	14.8%
Sweetened condensed	12.2%
Dried milk	38.7%
Skim Milk-	
Plain condensed	16.2%
Sweetened condensed	16.2%
Dried	52.1%
Sweet Cream	
Plain condensed	15.0%
Buttermilk-	
Sweetened condensed	15.0%
Dried	47.9%

Products like margarines and icecream are not straightforward. And descriptions often do not convey the presence of lactose, when they speak of 'whey' or 'emulsifiers'.

It is not always easy for a person with lactose intolerance to tell where lactose is to be found. They may not know it is inherent in whey used in infant formulae, or in icecream up to a level of 25% of the milk solids. They may not be aware that whey is used in less identifiable ways, as in sweets like caramel and fudge (which also may contain glucose syrup). They would not necessarily be mindful of powdered milk in bread. They may avoid foods they do not need to avoid, such as cheeses and creams of various varieties. Yet cheese is an excellent resource of balanced nutrition, retaining all the constituents of milk in concentrated form (being coagulated via lactic acid produced by bacteria, by adding rennet or other means).

Mostly such people are not very informed in their choices. They will avoid all chocolate although dark chocolate has quite a different balance of ingredients to milk chocolate, and may well prove quite acceptable. They may prefer cottage cheese to hard cheese, for other reasons like fat content, when actually the hard cheese would be preferable as cottage cheese is not fermented. They may choose soymilk preparations as an alternative, which could create new problems as I have mentioned earlier in this book, over and above any initial problem from the use of glucose syrup as a sweetener. They certainly do not make the kind of distinctions mentioned above, such as between skimmed milk in different guises and whole milk.

How much lactose can cause problems? Dr. Bayliss says that 25 gms of lactose will affect 92% of lactose intolerant adults. Some idea of what this means is given by the further statistic that a glass of whole milk will contain 12 gms. Dr. Bayliss emphasises that an individual is not usually wholly lactose intolerant. A person who cannot take a glass of milk or more at one sitting may well be able to take the same amount distributed throughout the day.

It has been thought that people with lactose intolerance would find milk acceptable, if it were hydrolysed to its monosaccharides, galactose and glucose. But I found myself at odds with this conclusion. My little grandson, Mark, reacted badly to just such milk in a special infant formula available here. And I had reacted unfavourably to galactose in my blind trial with sugars. Why we seemed different in this respect, and not in others, seemed a puzzle for which I had yet no answer.

I found myself at a parting of the ways on other points. The learned doctors made no mention in their book 'Lactose Digestion' of behaviour disorder in their list of symptoms produced by lactose intolerance. They mention stomach cramps, flatulence and diarrhoea produced by excess lactose passing into the colon, and not being digested properly there. But they are silent on other reactions familiar to us. Wakefulness and 'bad' behaviour that we had considered the likely result of hypoglycaemia. They mention the fact that lactose intolerance can give a flat blood glucose response, but do not analyse the implications of this.

They wrote nothing about 'super-heated' milk. I have already stated that we had traced cumulative bad reactions to the high percentage of dried milk powder in a gluten-free flour mix of Mauri Brothers and Thompson. We did not consider these were solely due to the higher percentage of lactose in that dried skimmed milk powder, because of previous experience with 'long-life' or superheated milk. My daughter, Vivian, had bought some cartons of 'long-life' milk for her two year old son to drink in Bali. He had become quite demented and hyperactive by the end of a week. Therefore the thought occurred to us that the powder used in the gluten-free mix might in fact be superheated. I spoke to the chemist at the manufacturer of that powder, Petersville. He admitted the milk was superheated, although not for long. I asked him what effect this might have. He thought none. Then I asked Professor Fraser. He had read an article somewhere which raised the possibility of distorted protein, which might conceivably have a toxic effect.

At the time, I wondered about the effect of heating on the lactose. I now found some, but not all, the answers in the book on

'Lactose Digestion'. There Dr. Rand states 'the common pasteurisation conditions employed for milk now avoid heating for such long times (30 to 60 minutes). The usual process is high temperature short time, in which the milk is heated to at least 72 degrees C and held for not less than 15 seconds. This is not sufficient time to accomplish lactose hydrolysis, which is a relatively slow process' (p. 221). Superheated milk is lifted to 85-96 degrees C, or just short of boiling, again for a short time (milk boils at 100 degrees). Whether the lactose is split into its monosaccharides in that short time at the higher heat, and that is the reason of our adverse reactions, I do not know. Perhaps it is due to another factor, like the jelling of the casein. We were more concerned with what it did, rather than what it was.

One thing was certain. I would have to take another hard look as to what the folk-wisdom was about combining milk with food. I came to some interesting conclusions.

First, our ancestors were not afraid of cream. They used a great deal more cream in recipes either with, or without, milk than we do today with our terror of fat and its effect in causing chloresterol, whether sweet cream in desserts, scones, rice puddings or pies, or sour cream with meat dishes or vegebles. This may have raised fat levels, but did not contribute to lactose levels.

Second, they used a great deal more 'cream' buttermilk than we do today with our preference for skimmed milk products.

Third, they used a considerable amount of cheese in various ways.

Fourth, they avoided boiling milk. They cooked milk long and slow. Custard in double boilers. Baked custards in the oven at very low temperatures. Dishes like rice puddings ditto.

Fifth, they ate butter in many ways where we now substitute margarine (with added powdered milk), or milk. They would put butter on their porridge at breakfast, in all baked products, and home-made sweets.

There is no doubt that concern for heart disease has tipped the balance towards low-fat milk products throughout a wide spectrum of foods, and therefore unfavourably to those with a low lactose tolerance. If statistics are correct, this would affect not merely ourselves, but nearly one third of any population group of British origin, particularly adults.

Now it remains for me to write a brief conclusion, summarising what our low maltose/glucose/lactose diet in fact is.

SOME RESEARCH ON PHYTIC ACID

In this discourse, I have emphasised the effect of phytic acid and other inhibitors in plant foodstuffs in impairing starch and protein digestion. It is worth pausing to quote some of the research on the subject to point up its relevance to maltose intolerance, which cannot be seen as a problem in isolation from dynamics of digestion as a whole.

In 1970, O'Dell and Savage suggested that the phytic acid in plant protein might account for the decreased availability of zinc in foods prepared from seeds. This report seemed amply justified in view of the numerous reports of impairment of zinc utilisation when phytate rich diets have been fed to different species e.g. chicks, pigs and rats.

One study showed reduced growth in rats, and a cyclic pattern of food intake characteristic of an uncomplicated zinc deficiency due to the presence of dietary phytate in a diet normally adequate with respect to zinc content. Growth was improved by increasing the dietary zinc concentration. (Davies and Nightingale Br. J. Nutrition 34 p. 243).

Another study tested breakfast cereals. They did not support the growth of rats. (Morris and Ellis Cereal Chemistry 58 (5) 303-6).

Yet another study showed that phytate ingested at the rate of 2.8 gms a day at 57% interfered with the bioavailability of divalent minerals, notably zinc, iron, calcium and magnesium. They concluded that reduction of phytic acid in the grain appeared prudent, especially because other sources of phytic acid, such as vegetable proteins, were being consumed in increasing amounts. (Tangkong et al. Cereal Chemistry 1981 58 pp. 347-50).

Results of balance studies were in general inconclusive until a team at the University of Berkeley did a stable isotope study of zinc absorption in four young men. They found that high levels of dietary phytate could result in zinc deficiency. (Am. J. Clin. Nutrition 1984 4 pp. 1071-9).

A team at the Shiraz University of Iran studied three men to determine whether high phytic acid from wholemeal bread could cause the disturbance of zinc and calcium metabolism prevalent among Iranian villagers. They analysed the effect of an intake of 2.5 grams of phytic acid daily in diets of unleavened compared to leavened bread. They found the higher phytic acid caused the plasma calcium and serum phosphorus to fall and stay there, the nitrogen balance to decrease, a negative calcium balance to persist, and the composition of the blood to alter. Susceptibility differed between the three men. They concluded that 'alteration to the composition of blood while phytate was being ingested indicate that losses of zinc, iron and calcium were large enough to have generalised effects.

They also noticed that inhibition of yeast phytase enzymes, which could split the phytic acid, occurred in the presence of wholemeal, but thought this was due to other inhibitors, and not to calcium. (Rheingold et al. Lancet 1973 p. 283).

However, it should be noted these conclusions were qualified by a further study to explain why an intake of added purified phytic acid was less effective in decreasing retention of zinc and calcium than an intake of equivalent amounts occurring naturally in wholemeal bread. They examined other constituents of wholemeal flour as possible metal binding agents. They concluded that the cellulose, hemicellulose and lignin of fibre (bran) interferes with metal absorption simply by stimulating the peristaltic action, and thus increasing the rate of passage through the digestive tract. The meals thereby become bound to these indigestible fibre compounds, and remain unavailable for gastro-intestinal consumption.

The same team assessed the opposite effect in an experiment with rats- whether yeast fermentation in bread modified the effect of phytic acid. In fact, fermentation modified the phytic acid far more effectively than expected from the relatively moderate destruction of phytic acid during the action of the yeast leaven.

Another study in 1980 showed that the greater the addition of yeast, the more the phytic acid reduction in breads, whether rye, wholemeal or white; but four hours fermentation was necessary for substantial reduction. (Harland and Harland. Br. Nutrition J. 1980 41 p. 591).

Tang et al showed that the hydrolysis of phytic acid slowed down after two hours with little additional loss up to five hours. It was thought enzymatic action had ceased. (Cereal Chemistry 1981 58 p. 231).

If concentrations of calcium phytase, or phosphatase, are added to yeast, they are capable of reducing the concentration of phytate to 1/3 or 1/8 of its original value. Storage at room temperature for up to 96 hours further reduced it. (Knorr and

Carlson J. Food Science 46 pp. 1866-9). The figure was lowest for barley, oats and yellow corn.

A test of twenty breads with added bran, both raw and cooked, and with leavening times of 0-120 hours was made with 42 students. They proved that the phytic acid in bran is reduced by fermentation, and the amount of zinc absorbed grows as each fermentation is prolonged. (Novert and Sandstrom J. Nutrition 1985 47 p. 53).

Studies in Egypt, Pakistan and Iran supported the conclusion of the Dublin National Nutrition survey in World War 2 that calcium deficiency was greater in diets where more unfermented or unleavened bread, than fermented or leavened, wholegrain bread was eaten, significantly in populations which had plenty of Vitamin D from sunlight.

Studies with rice are less common, although half the world's population lives on rice. A comparative study on unpolished vs polished rice was carried out in Ceylon in 1950. Twelve normal males were given 9 oz. of raw rice equivalent to 27 oz of cooked rice, for four weeks. On unpolished rice there was a substantial decrease in the metabolic balance of calcium and magnesium in six of the subjects, and a negative balance in six. The excretion rate was increased. On polished rice, this balance changed to positive with a decreased excretion, although the actual intake of calcium was less. The team concluded 'this obviously suggests that, from the point of view of calcium metabolism, polished rice is to be preferred.' But they qualified this finding by saying that moderately polished rice gave a better calcium and magnesium balance than highly polished. (Cullumbine et al. Br. J. of Nutrition 1950 4 p. 101). The brands that qualify best on the Australian market are Sungold and Uncle Bens.

Researchers perceived they needed a measure by which zinc adequacy or otherwise in the diet could be measured in terms of the presence or absence of zinc. In 1975, a scientist called Oberleas devised a formula known as the phytate-zinc molar ratio. This was a technical formula of the ratio of millimoles of phytate per serving to millimoles of zinc. These were calculated by dividing the milligrams of phytic acid by 660 and the milligrams of zinc by 65.4 (the atomic weight of zinc). Using this formula, he arrived at a kind of 'Plimsoll Line' for zinc deficiency in man.

When a diet contained phytate, and had a phytate-zinc molar ratio of 15+, inhibition of zinc absorption, similar to that seen in rats and chickens, might result. (Oberleas J. Nutrition 1980 110 pp. 1037-45).

Ratios of 12+ reduced growth in rats, and uptake of zinc in the liver. Such ratios were common in modern self-selected diets, which were rarely adequate in zinc. They were even more common in vegetarian meals, the ratio of a typical vegetarian meal being 23 to 1. The diets of Trappist monks are even higher with their exclusion of meat or eggs.

The zinc status at the time of absorption of phytate is important. As one of the predominant sources of minimally reduced phytic acid in western diet today is breakfast cereals, biochemists have been concerned as to whether their consumption is creating levels of phytic acid that are likely to threaten a serious imbalance of mineral nutrition.

Davies measured the phytic acid content of twelve high-fibre cereals and granola products. They varied from ready-to-eat cereals, to old fashioned quick-cooking, or instant products; all with added bran, sunflower seeds, nuts, dried fruits, and other minimally processed ingredients, depending on the product. He found that the percentage of phytic acid was not significantly different by cereal group, indicating no consistent effect from processing, or lack of processing, by cereals. What was important was that the phytate-zinc molar ratio of all of them was higher than the 6:1 thought necessary to prevent zinc depletion.

This finding cannot be ignored in view of another report that intake of phytic acid increases as intake of dietary fibre from whole grains, fruits, nuts and vegetables is increased (Harland and Prosky Cereal Chemistry 1979 58 (4) pp. 347-350).

To comment briefly on the question of phytate effect in creating iron deficiency (iron being required for red blood cells and the proper function of certain enzymes), it is now generally agreed that it is poorly available from phytate rich foods- whether cereals, legumes or nuts- unless they are eaten with iron rich foods such as meat and eggs, or with a good protagonist such as citric acid, found in orange, lemon, lime, grapefruit and pawpaw.

This conclusion that a nutritional deficiency of zinc, calcium, and iron (as of copper, manganese and magnesium) can occur under appropriate dietary conditions, depending on which first becomes limiting in the diet, unless careful complementation is made, has serious implications for diet. (Cereal Chemistry 59 (3) p. 257). It has particular implication for a family like mine, owing to the fact that manganese is important for normal glucose utilisation,

98

and calcium is vital for the activity, and maximum stability, of alpha-amylase in starch digestion.

Phytic acid is reduced under certain conditions.

A. *PREPARATION AND COOKING*

1. Milling of wholegrains from wholemeal to white flour removes 35-88% of the phytic acid according to the degree of milling in stripping off the bran.

2. Boiling encourages leaching of both water and acid extractable acid, as tested in three legumes (Aust. Food Reports 1982 28 p. 43).

3. Autoclaving at over 116 degrees removes 50-80% of the phytic acid depending on the length of cooking (Talbekia & Link 1980 p. 40).

B. *ACTIVATING INHERENT ENZYMES*

Phytase is an enzyme present in most seeds, plants and in the intestine of animals including man. It becomes active with moisture and heat, as exemplified below.

1. Soaking at temperatures between 45 and 60 degrees (-salt). Results are variable according to the amount of inherent phytase. The scale of response runs - wheat and rye 45 and 60 minutes respectively, barley 7 hours, rice 8 hours, and oats 12 hours. Beans fall in between. Figures for soya bean and sweet potato are similar. Hydrolysis slows down after two hours with little additional loss up to 5 hours when enzymatic action seems to cease. (Tang et al. Cereal Chemistry 1981 58 p. 231).

2. Fermentation at 45-60 degrees reduces phytic acid (Rheingold Cereal Chemistry 1975 57 p. 366). More phytic acid is hydrolysed with yeast than water. The figure was lowest for barley, oats and yellow corn (Daniells & Fisher Cereal Chemistry 1981 p. 461).

Clearly a growing body of evidence by biochemists over the past fifty years seems to indicate that far from bran (fibre) being valuable in diet, as so enthusiastically claimed on all sides, the reverse may be the case. Although nutrients are indeed theoretically present in larger amounts in wholemeal flour than in white flour, brown rather than white rice, and so on, it does not follow they are also absorbed in the body in large amounts since the phytic acid combines with zinc, calcium and iron to form insoluble salts. Moreover the roughage in itself which has no inherent food value apart from these trace elements, leads to peristalsis (more violent contractions of the gut to aid motility of food) and decreased absorption. In fact the very processing, which causes the loss of nutrients so strongly condemned by health enthusiasts, may in fact enhance the biological value of the residual endosperm flour.

What exactly is fibre? Fibre consists of those plant constituents which are resistant to digestion by the secretions of the human gastro-intestinal tract. The diverse chemical compounds of fibre (not uniform for all plants) include cellulose and hemicellulose (effective bulk producers that may be as high as 60%), mucilages, waxes, pectins, gums and lignins.

The foregoing facts give pause for thought in view of the fact the medical profession still strongly advises increasing fibre in our diet as good for our health in general, and insurance against a variety of serious diseases, colon, cancer, diabetes, and heart in particular. The virtue of fibre is said to lie in its ability to provide bulk in digestion, and the fact it moves through the small intestine, to be digested in the large intestine. Moreover, it contains the highest proportion of the vitamins and minerals, particularly in cereals.

This advice ignores the fact that the whole grains may be rich in vital components of the diet, but these components may not necessarily be biologically available because of the existence of inhibitors and antagonists of various kinds. It does not take account of the fact that starch is capable of producing the same effect in the gastro-intestinal tract as foods which are rich in fibre, when food is partly gelatinised in cooking or processing. And, interestingly enough, pregelatinised starch is used widely in supermarket foods such as instant gravies, sauces, soups, spoonable desserts, jelly beans, gum drops and so forth.

In this context, I quote Frolich. 'For a long time, it was believed that starch was completely digested and absorbed in the small intestine of human beings because of the presence of starch hydrolysing enzymes (alpha-amylase) in the pancreatic secretions that will hydrolyse starch to maltose, maltotriose and dextrins, and disaccharidases in the intestinal wall that will hydrolyse further to free glucose.' (Procdgs. Symp. R.A. Chemical Institute 1987).

Indeed it is possible that significant amounts of starch are not completely absorbed, the amount depending on protein or lipid interactions with the starch. The ease of digestion is facilitated both by heat processing and fermentation. It has been demonstrated, at least in the case of wheat, that the starch of

100

wheat is only completely absorbed in the small intestine if the protein is removed (N. England J. Med 304 pp. 891-2). If intact, 20% of the starch was malabsorbed.

It is clear that the constant emphasis on whole grain cereals, or whole foods, in diet ignores the adverse effects in favour of the asssumed beneficial effects. It also ignores a number of studies which show that high-fibre diets with their indigestible polysaccharides cause a significant decrease in apparent protein digestibility by exerting a considerable influence upon the activities of proteolytic digestive enzymes in the small intestine.

A resume of studies on the subject says 'although the mechanism by which pancreatic enzyme adaptation to diet composition is not clearly understood, dietary fibre appears to affect the excretion of digestive enzymes, especially proteolytic enzymes, through its inhibitory capacity against the enzymes.' (Cereal Chemistry 60 (4) 1983 p.262).

One biochemist insists his study of fibre led him to take a very qualified view of the subject. 'Claims made for increased dietary fibre to prevent, or cure, diseases, need to be substantiated by extended clinical studies' (Kunara Cereal Food World Jan. 1977 p. 1619).

This view has already been urged by the Irish National Survey 1940-42 into rickets in children, repeated by a Scottish team reassessing their work. 'The Irish National Survey warns against the uncritical advocacy of the consumption of wholemeal and high fibre diets, particularly at times of rapid growth. Children and women on such diets, particularly where ultra-violet exposure is limited by latitude, or urban environment, or social custom, should be protected by Vitamin D supplements' (Br. J. Nutrition 45 p. 17).

Much of the research, from which I have quoted, tends to validate the conclusion I had reached separately, that plant food in its raw state is basically hostile to man. Food is better well prepared for cooking than not prepared at all. Food is better cooked than raw. When food is cooked, some methods are preferable to others. Facts known to our ancestors for many centuries. Facts that must invalidate any presumption that the closer to 'natural' food the better.

My own experience tended to validate it in that I had had a clear watershed of change at the University from diet based on folk wisdom to diet based on the theory that whole grains were healthier. I was resident at the Womens College when the Council appointed their first dietitian in residence. She changed everything from what might be said to have been traditional 'boarding-school' type diet to the new fashionable 'health' diet. This change had precipitated a total decline in my physical and mental health, and my University performance. The worse I became in the next decade the more I ate health foods thinking to cure myself, all the while creating a vicious circle of decline until my gastric, allergic, energy fluctuation, fatigue, and inability to concentrate were incapacitating. Only when I abolished all symptoms by moving in the opposite direction from health foods to highly refined foodstuffs, did I understand what a fragile dynamic balance exists between bad or good health. In our case this depended on abandoning any absolute approach to foodstuffs, and considering food always as a dynamic, acceptable in one guise, but not in another. I quote two of our most common articles of diet, tea and coffee, by way of example.

I had supposed once that coffee was the same, whether consumed as instant or percolated coffee. In terms of the phytate/zinc molar ratio, Harland and Oberleas demonstrated this is by no means so. They studied both phytate and zinc concentrations in four instant coffee brands, and seven percolated brands. They found that the total phytate of instant coffee (all brands) was less than 50% of percolated (all brands), while the concentration of zinc was four times greater. Therefore instant coffee had a far better phytate/zinc molar ratio than percolated coffee. Since some of these ratios were higher than ten, they concluded they could affect the health of the inveterate coffee drinker, who consumes several cups of coffee a day. The stronger the coffee, the worse (J. Food Science 50 pp. 832-3). It was suggested the difference was due to the fact that the whole bean is consumed in instant coffee with the compensating minerals such as zinc, copper and manganese present, whereas only that part of the bean which drains out with hot water is consumed in percolated coffee.

The same research team found the opposite true of tea. Instant tea had four times the phytic acid than brewed tea; but there was little difference between brands compared to coffee. It is worthy of note that the phytic acid was still high, although the processing of tea from green to brown would counteract such anti-nutrients to some extent.

However, diet is not simply a matter of the balance of components from the one plant resource. It is important to remember in this context that trace element nutrition can be modified or enhanced by the presence, or lack, of other trace minerals, and dietary components. And that copper, iron and zinc- three of the most vital trace elements- are better absorbed from animal than plant sources, that is from meat, fish and milk or milk products. Therefore some article of diet from these three groups should be included with every meal, including breakfast.

As some indication of just how important these three minerals are even in minute amounts, I will summarise their functions.

Zinc is required for at least twenty enzyme systems, including those regulating Vitamin A metabolism, nucleic acid metabolism, protein synthesis, and behaviour patterns. It is required for cell growth, and hormone levels for normal growth. It detoxifies toxic trace elements such as cadmium and lead.

Iron is required in fairly high amounts for red blood corpuscles.

Copper is required for iron metabolism, and cross-linking of the amino acid, lysine, in the protein collagen- the major portion holding all the cells of the body together- the protein on which bone mineral is deposited, the protein which forms tendons and ligaments.

Other trace elements are also crucial to enzyme systems. Nickel is required for DNA metabolism, and cell membranes. Selenium acts against cancer and heavy metal poisoning. Vanadium is required for growth, and perhaps for the control of the cholesterol concentration in the blood. Tin is needed for normal growth. The requirements of silicon are as yet unknown.

At least three more are of particular importance to those, such as members of my family, with specific carbohydrate intolerance. Chromium is necessary for normal carbohydrate metabolism, in that it acts as a glucose tolerance factor. It also counteracts serum chloresterol. Calcium is required for activity and stability of alpha-amylase in starch digestion. And last, but not least, manganese is required for normal glucose utilisation, lactose synthesis, and oxidation (although magnesium can substitute). It is also essential for cartilage, (tendon and bone structure), and the central nervous system.

Because trace elements are said to be high in the bran of cereals, and in milk, and a maltose/glucose/lactose intolerance diet excludes any cereal bran, and reduces milk, it is extremely important for anyone on such a diet to ensure a steady intake of animal and fish protein or cheese at all meals, and to increase intake of alternative starches.

103

ALTERNATIVE FLOURS

As wheat is such an important resource of carbohydrate in western society, and, to a lesser extent, its allied cereals, rye, oats, barley and millet, the first reaction of anyone told they cannot eat these cereals, except to a limited degree, is dismay. A consternation echoed by observers. What can you eat, they cry non-plussed? Such a response shows how meagre in variety our diet has become, how lacking in imagination we have become.

Quite a few products on the market provide alternatives, some of them pre-processed such as packet instant puddings, corn and potato chips, or Chinese rice noodles. Quite a few recipes offer attractive meals with other starches, such as corn, sweet potato, taro, and sago.

Corn is quite widely used as a staple of diet in America, particularly South America, and Africa. The other three, though now a common article of diet in western countries, are indispensable items of diet in Asia and the Pacific.

CORN

Corn is an unexplained enigma in the context of a maltose intolerance diet. Theoretically, I would presume that it must be banished along with wheat, as it is equally a producer of glucose syrup. But in fact, it does not appear to cause the far-reaching disturbance, as wheat does, to our physiology. We do not consume it daily, of course, as people do in other parts of the world. But even that fact does not account for the difference; a difference that is important to us, as corn is readily available in our society, and offers an easy alternative carbohydrate resource in our diet.

The consumption of corn is being widely extended in many countries of the world for animal as well as human feed. Corn is one of the best sources of metabolisable energy being readily digested, having low levels of anti-nutrients such as trypsin and chymotrypsin inhibitors. It has high dietary fibre levels. It has all the important vitamins except Vitamin B12. It is a good source of Vitamins A and E and carotene. Its oil is highly polyunsaturated, and is rich in linoleic acid, which aids absorption of saturated fats, and fat-soluble nutrients.

Corn has disadvantages, but these are only important if it is a daily staple in diet. Its niacin (Vitamin B3) is unavailable unless the corn is processed with lime or dilute alkali. Its protein is deficient in the amino acids lysine and tryptophan, so that a complement of soybean protein which has a high percentage of both is important. It is low in calcium compared to other grains. Eighty per cent of its phosphorus is in the form of phytic acid, none of which is milled with the bran as with wheat, while its trace mineral content is low compared to small grains. Therefore, it is advisable in a diet high in corn to include supplementary sources of the trace minerals, including zinc, iron, manganese, copper and iodine to prevent deficiencies. (n.b. selenium is highly toxic at a level not much higher than normal requirement).

Corn is most familiar in western countries these days as cornflour, corn chips, tortillas, taco shells, cornchips or cornflakes. In the Americas it is also commonly eaten as corn meal in corn bread, muffins, fritters, and as corn grits; or as polenta, either fine or coarse. Corn breakfast foods, and cornmeal are often fortified with supplementary vitamins.

However, corn is often consumed in a less obvious way as cornflour or glucose syrup. The first is used as a binder in processed meats, and in packaged dry mixes such as batters and pancakes. The second is used in a wide variety of other foods such as drinks, tinned fruit, confectionery, icecream, baked goods, and salad dressings.

The use of corn as a sweetener demands more explanation than the rest as the end result is not so readily identified as other corn products.

The conversion of starch to sugar began during the Napoleonic Wars when the French were cut off from their West Indian supplies of sugar by an English blockade. Before long, ways of hydrolysing starch to sugar were found. A range of corn syrups was ultimately developed with an index known as DE from 20 to 99.4. Although all are referred to as glucose syrups, the actual level of D glucose may be very low. The higher the DE the more the dextrose, the lower the DE the more the malto-dextrins. The higher the DE the sweeter.

These glucose syrups are not merely used because they are a substitute for the sweetness of sugar. They are also used for a range of other properties which are amazingly various. They are used as dispersing agents in synthetic coffee whiteners; moisture holding agents in breads, pastries and meats; for sweetness, body, and osmotic pressure in beverages and wines; for coating strength, hardness, colour and gloss in chewing gum and candies; for colour and flavour in crusts in bread, and strength for slicing and handling; for texture in icecream and cakes. The list goes on endlessly, as any

105

supermarket shelves will testify to anyone who bothers to read the labels.

SWEET POTATO

The sweet potato is not closely related to the common potato, so long familiar to the west, although it also originated in America where it was widely distributed in the tropics before its global diffusion after 1492. It is not the root of a ground plant, but the tuberous root of a perennial vine.

Unlike the potato, its leaves as well as its root are eaten in some parts of the world such as Indonesia. Like the potato, it has a highly digestible carbohydrate. But it has even more calories, and appreciable quantities of ascorbic acid and minerals. The protein of sweet potato, which varies from 5-23% depending on the level of the fertiliser, has a higher lysine level than rice or wheat flour, so its addition to either of these, whether as vegetable or flour, gives an enhanced human nitrogen balance.

It is not considered edible raw, even for animals. Taiwanese farmers cook it before giving it to pigs as feed. Experiments with rats showed that, if it was preheated, they had an enhanced nitrogen retention and balance, had a better growth rate, and lived longer.

There are three types of sweet potato- orange, white and purple- with a range of levels for many nutrients. Orange sweet potato contains higher calcium, magnesium and Vitamin A, but a lower level of organic acids. White sweet potato contains lower Vitamin C and niacin. Purple sweet potato contains higher niacin and starch, and lower levels of disaccharides.

Sweet potatoes are mainly used as a vegetable in the West with a wider range of use than white potato, due to its capacity to combine well with fruit and fruit flavours like orange marmalade. They can also be made into acceptable chips, and flakes, like white potatoes, but these are not yet readily available in the West. Nor is sweet potato flour, which can be used for baking in bread, and biscuits with other flours.

WHITE POTATO

White potatoes are one of the most important food crops in the world. They became central articles of food diet in colder countries, such as Ireland, and Northern Europe after its importation into Europe by Sir Walter Raleigh, because it weathered the cold climate better than cereals. But potato flour from potatoes has never been as widely used in Western European cuisine as in central and Northern Europe.

Potatoes are an extremely versatile source of carbohydrate bulk in diet due to their capacity to blend with other flavours such as cheese, or herbs, or to complement other foods such as pumpkin, carrots, parsnips, onions or meat. This versatility is enhanced today by food technology with the popular chips, either packaged or fresh from take away shops. They are a valuable source of retrograde starch due to the fact they are often cooled and reheated in casseroles, potato cakes and other dishes; and the fact they gelatinise easily with their large particle structure. They are usually cooked at high temperatures, often for long intervals. This helps to nullify any anti-nutrients present.

TARO

Taro is worth far more consideration than it has been given by those who are allergic or intolerant of wheat, or intolerant of milk. It is superior to other starchy staples. The size of the granule is small (1/10th that of potato), and it is almost totally digestible (97%) with efficient release of nutrients during digestion. For this reason it is used extensively for infant formulae in America, and as a starting product for baby weaning in Samoa.

It has several advantages. Its vitamin content is higher than that of sago or rice, particularly of Vitamin A. It is low in fat. It is high in riboflavin and niacin, and relatively high in calcium, phosphate and potassium. Its protein level is adequate to maintain health in adults, but supplementation is necessary for growing children or pregnant mothers. It is a relatively poor source of ascorbic acid and carotene.

Taro is eaten widely in Africa and Asia. In the Pacific it is of supreme importance in the diet. Both the tuber and leaves are eaten, but only after peeling and soaking, drying and cooking, preferably to a high temperature, owing to the presence of an acrid agent capable of a toxic effect. This appears to be a proteolytic enzyme similar to trypsin. A positive correlation between removal of acridity from the raw taro and weight gain has been noted.

Taro is consumed in a variety of ways in countries where it is a staple. Its corms are roasted or fried (in the Phillipines), boiled (as in Indian curries), baked or steamed (in the South Pacific). They are made into a fresh or fermented purplish-grey paste called poi, popular in Hawaii. Taro is consumed as chips (like potato chips);

as grits for breakfast foods; as flakes in puddings, purees, icecreams or drinks; as flour in a cereal base or for sweet desserts.

A related tuber called dasheen is eaten in Indonesia, which is locally known as 'elephant's ear'. These are nutty in flavour, and contain more carbohydrates and proteins than the potato.

A nation like Australia, based in the heartland of the Pacific, might profitably experiment even more widely with some of the starchy foods common in that region than it is already doing. Sweet potato is already widely available in all varieties, but not yet as a flour. Taro is available in very limited outlets, but only as a vegetable, not as chips or flour. Tapioca flour has recently come on the market as well as the long-familiar tapioca beads of traditional European desserts.

CASSAVA (TAPIOCA)

Cassava is the potato of the East. However, its protein and fat are inferior to that of either potatoes or rice, since it is basically a starch. This nutritional deficiency can be balanced if it is combined with soy. The combined quality of bread made from tapioca flour and defatted soybean flour is of good quality, and nutritionally better than wheat for bread, biscuits and cakes.

There are two varieties of the cassava plant- bitter and sweet. The bitter is highly poisonous when fresh, and must be cooked to destroy the poison (prussic acid) and cannot be eaten fresh. The sweet is perfectly harmless. The leaves and shoots are eaten as a vegetable, high in proteins and vitamins. The tuber is used in a variety of ways either as a flour, or in beads- boiled, steamed, baked, fried, or fermented.

It is basically a starch that can be used like other starches for baked and gelatinised products. A bread can be made of it in combination with soya flour, but will have a cake rather than a bread crumb. The problem is, of course, the lack of gluten, which gives cereal its swelling property. A binding agent must be added during the preparation of the dough to bind the starch granules, such as egg white, gum, or glyceryl monostereate.

The cassava starch is well prepared to make it palatable and digestible. It is washed, peeled, rasped and strained. The resulting flour is further processed to make the familiar tapioca flakes or pearls by highly skilled workers, who moisten, heat and stir the flour until the starch agglomerates into the semi-translucent white balls which have such high keeping qualities that they have always been a stock item in every western food

108

pantry. When cooked, these tapioca pellets produce clear, tender flavourless gels favoured as a thickening agent in puddings, fruits, pies, and soups not only in domestic cooking, but also industrial plants.

Tapioca's absorbent capacity is seen by the fact that 1/4 cup will thicken 1 pint of fluid.

ARROWROOT

The only genuine arrowroot comes from the West Indies. It is the starch residue from repeated washing of the grated peeled root of the arrowroot plant. It yields a fine transparent, odourless and pleasant tasting jelly in boiling water; and has long been a thickening agent for both savoury and sweet dishes in the West and for biscuits and blancmanges. It is also valued as an invalid food on account of its highly digestible quality. Other starches are sold as arrowroot, as for example from cassava. They are all basically starch with little mineral value.

SAGO

This food starch is distinctive in that it derives from the pith of the sago palm, native to Indonesia. It must be harvested before the palm develops a flower spike at the end of 15 years.

The pith is ground into a flour, and strained. Like tapioca, it can be used either as a flour, or further processed into the beads better known in the West than the flour.

It is used mostly in puddings in Great Britain, boiled with milk with or without eggs, fruit juice or flavoured water. It is used in fruit puddings and soups in Germany and Scandinavia, and for sauce or thickening agent for soups.

BUCKWHEAT FLOUR

This is not a true cereal, but a member of the rhubarb family. The proteins are not gluten-like, and are suitable for gluten-free diets. It has the essential amino acids, including lysine, arginine and glycine. It also has high fibre and a distinctive taste.

It is commonly used in the diet of Eastern Europe and parts of the U.S.S.R. for making cakes and pancakes (blinis), and in the U.S.A. as a cereal food.

RICE

Rice has played a prominent part in Western diet for many centuries. When wheat flour was still scarce and dear in Great

Britain, rice flour was often added in bread making. It is still valued as an ingredient of bread for the fact that it helps to keep it moist. Rice or ground rice, however, were more commonly used as desserts than for savoury dishes in Western diets until modern times. Rice flour (which is finer than ground rice) is creeping back into favour in the West for those on wheat-free diets, though in former days it was widely used under the name 'cornflour' in many recipes.

The various varieties have different virtues. Long grain rices remain more easily separated on cooking. Short grain rices are more glutinous and more likely to adhere. This word refers to the property of stickiness, and has no link with the word for grain protein 'gluten'. Of the short grain rices, pearl rice is the most glutinous of all, and generally used for cakes and sweets. Short grain rice is, of course, used for breakfast cereal products like rice bubbles, and puffed rice. Ground rice is used in puddings and rice biscuits and snacks. Rice is probably one of the most valuable and versatile of foods known to man. It is high in protein, and very low in fat. It has the amazing capacity to blend with almost any flavour, sweet or sour, and therefore appears in a bewildering variety of dishes.

SOYBEAN FLOUR

It is important to deal with soyflour at greater length, as the high quality and fraction of its protein makes it a vital supplement to all the refined flours usually used in substitution for wheat flour in a great many Western recipes.

Soybeans are one of the five sacred foods in China, which include rice, barley, millet and wheat. In the east, men have long valued them for their benefit to the function of heart, liver and kidneys; and for the health and endurance of their animals. In the West at first they were more commonly fed to animals, but have been gaining favour as human food.

But in both regions of the world it has long been recognised that soybeans must be processed before they can be eaten because of anti-nutritional factors. In the East, this is effected often by more than one process- drying, heating, fermenting, curing. In America, the process used exposes the bean to moisture, heat and hexane (purified petroleum hydrocarbons). Such process demands a high tonnage and constant operation of the plant.

Smaller plants with less adequate processing are found more commonly in England and elsewhere. Their major concern is

110

simply to prevent rancidity and bitterness, not to remove anti-nutrients. Indeed, they err on the conservative side in heat-treatment to avoid reducing the appeal of the soyflour by darkening its colour. The lack of a consistent standard in a comparison of soyflours from three different sources in Europe, undertaken in the Nutrition Department of Cork University College, showed a significant difference between the three- a fact of importance to infant feeding in alternative-to-milk formulae. This fact makes it difficult to draw conclusions from feeding trials involving commercial soybean products, unless the processing history of those used is known. Suffice to say that most soyflour processing plants in small countries like Australia would produce soyflour so lightly processed as to raise some doubts whether adverse biologically active compounds present in the raw soybeans have been adequately neutralised. Certainly my eldest daughter, Rosalind, found a high level of local soyflour in cakes, pancakes etc. (50-50%) caused serious digestive disturbance.

Modern research with chicks, rats and mice, have demonstrated that raw, untreated meal can stimulate hypersecretion of pancreatic enzymes, depress metabolisable energy of the diet, enlarge the pancreas, and lower glycogen levels in liver and muscle. It can also reduce fat absorption and inhibit growth.

The adverse factors are thought to be some 7-10 trypsin inhibitors (accounting for between 30-60% of the inhibiting properties of the raw meal), multiple hemoglutinins, phytic acid (twice as much as in most cereals, though the levels can vary), and goitrogens. All these are heat sensitive. Good results ensue from autoclaving 15-20 minutes (steam 30). Soybean meal diets require added mineral and vitamins unless there are alternative complementary sources of protein, particularly because the level of the two amino acids which can limit growth of young humans and animals in excess, lysine and tryptophan, are higher than in common cereals. An ideal combination is with corn, the resulting corn/soy mixture being greatly superior to either alone.

The adverse factors are well known in the Orient where soybeans in most soybean products have been subject to careful preparation. Tofu in Indonesia, for example, is subject to four different processes. One study showed that phytic acid was not effectively abolished until the end of the last process. In this context, it is important to remember that the concentration of phytic acid is much higher in soybean protein isolates than in soyflour. Therefore soy drinks and other foods based on protein isolate have to be treated with even more caution as to whether they are really the valuable health food they claim to be; particularly when glucose syrup is used to sweeten them.

Given that soybeans must be seen in the context of the whole diet, they have inherent advantages. They are a good source of Vitamin B complex (80% as potent as cows' milk). Their protein levels are three times higher than in rice, corn or oats, being intermediate in value between animals and plants. The amino acids are 65-100% available, if the soybean flour has been subjected to proper heat treatment, and approximate to cows' milk, though requiring a methionine supplement. They contain both water-soluble and fat-soluble vitamins. Their B carotene (the biological precursor of Vitamin A) is half that of cows' milk.

One of the main disadvantages of soybeans is that the availability of most minerals is quite low compared to cereals, due to the fact that the bean has twice as much phytic acid as most cereals. Another is that it is a poor source of Vitamin C, lower in iodine, chlorine and proteinase activity than most cereals, and virtually devoid of Vitamin D and Vitamin B12.

This discussion on the need to know the origin of soyflour is more pertinent now than it was a generation ago in view of the many concealed uses of soyflour. It is being used quite extensively in manufactured foods such as meat extenders in various sausages and pies; in soups, beverages and desserts; and as a supplement for cereals in breads, and pastries.

WHEAT AND ALTERNATIVE STARCH

The unique factor that singles wheat out from any other foodstuff is its gluten protein. It only exists to a much smaller degree in similar cereals from which breads have been made, namely barley, and rye, or in oats. None of these make satisfactory breads in their own right. It does not exist at all in corn, rice, or any of the tubers already mentioned.

Gluten found in wheat has the ability to stretch and retain gases produced by yeast or other leavening agents in a host of tiny air bubbles, which form the basic structures of bread. The quality and quantity of this gluten protein determines the loaf volume. The higher the better. The type of wheat, whether hard or soft, governs the water absorption capacity of the flour, the hard wheat absorbing more and therefore proving more economical.

Bread has four basic ingredients. Flour, yeast, salt and water, with a number of optional additions such as flour bleaching agents, fats, milk products, sugars, bread improvers, emulsifiers and preservatives. The flour is mixed with water, kneaded, turned and folded, to trap the air in the gluten. When the sticky mass turns into a dry smooth dough, it is left to rise, then punched down to rise a second time. This was a straight dough method. It is now seldom used commercially, because it is a time-dependent system which cannot be used for large batches. Moreover it has an uneven grain, and is chewier than bread produced by the modern sponge-dough system.

The sponge dough method is very rapid. The sponge consists of flour water, yeast and yeast food which ferments for 4-5 hours before the flour is added. The yeast food consists of a variety of bread improvers, the purpose of them all being the same- to speed up the process which once took a leisurely few hours. Like most technical changes in the food industry, this change has been made because it offers some benefits to the technician. Not only is the mixing time shorter, but the resultant dough is more tolerant to variation in time schedule, and the bread has a more consistent texture for cutting as for sandwiches. Indeed, the bulk of sliced, wrapped bread from commercial factories, made on the instant dough principle, takes about ninety minutes from start to finish.

The low protein wheat used for ordinary domestic uses in cakes, etc., and the durum hard wheats used for pasta making or semolina, are not relevant to this discussion, which is only concerned with the need for a maltose intolerant diet. Therefore it does not include anything but white bread flour, not even wholemeal, despite the fact people throughout the world have been urged to consume wholemeal rather than white flour on the grounds that the vitamins and minerals are higher in the wholemeal.

It is important to state that this difference between wholemeal and white flour is not as drastic as once thought. The content of most B vitamins, except thiamin, increases slightly in the white flour. The Vitamin B3 is not bound as it is in the wholemeal. The minerals are also more biologically available. And the digestibility of the white 'low-extraction' flour is higher. White flour is commonly fortified in any case to counteract any diminished effect.

In the days when bread was made at a slow pace, and left to rise all night, it is possible the slow fermentation at a warm

113

temperature may have effectively diminished any adverse factors in wholemeal flour. But this cannot be the case today, where such cottage bakery methods are never employed.

They may also have been reduced by the use of other foodstuffs such as potatoes, or rice. Mashed potato was often combined with wheat flour, in the proportion of 4 to 1 (rubbed in like fat), in times of grain shortage or financial stringency. It required more salt than for ordinary bread, and a lower temperature for baking. It was said to make a very light, moisture-retentive loaf ideal for toast, easier to spread. Rice bread used boiled rice, in the proportion of 3 ozs (3/4 cup in 11/2 cup of water) to just over 1 lb of flour, mixed into the flour while still warm. The variety of rice is not important, but the proportion given is for white rice. The rice bread is moist, delicious and ideal for sandwiches. The Greeks make a rice bread known as orinde, which is prized.

Both potato and rice flour are used to dust bread dough at the moulding stage, particularly fat-enriched doughs. They dry the surface of the dough without sticking.

These days recipes for 6-hour-long doughs are hard to come by. Most books give shorter times, and therefore the recipes are useless because the time factor governs the balance of the essential ingredients. The bakers who still know the time-honoured methods are hard to find.

OATS

Oats are very low in gluten compared to wheat. They have similar anti-nutrients, including phytic acid, but no inherent phytase which can be activated by soaking or germination to remove the latter. They also contain maltose, as wheat does, and therefore are unacceptable in any of their common forms in modern diet such as rolled oats, muesli, or hulled flour. Now oatmeal was central to British diet for many centuries, along with barley, when such wheat as was grown was exported, and only available to the rich, and when oats was easier to grow, thriving on poorer soils than wheat, and proving easier to keep.

It is intriguing to learn that oats were not always eaten unfermented, as recipes handed down would appear to suggest. Modern books which give recipes for the famous Scotch or Yorkshire oatcakes say nothing about fermentation, but it would seem that these flat, griddle-baked bannocks were often made with a natural or sour leavening. The fine and medium oatmeal flours were generally used for making oatcakes. These oatcakes keep a long time without deteriorating. Oatmeal muffins were also leavened, while a porridge called 'sowens' was fermented.

As the level of gluten is ten times less in oats than in wheat, it is likely that the incidence of frank coeliac disease was lower, when oatmeal was the staple food of Britain, than today when wheat has displaced oats to become the primary food. For this very reason, it has been thought that mild coeliacs can tolerate gluten.

Before leaving this subject of gluten tolerance, I should define coeliac disease to distinguish it from the profile of maltose intolerance, which shares an inability to handle wheat.A person with coeliac disease suffers a toxic response to eating wheat, localised in the small intestine. Mature absorptive epithelial cells are destroyed on the villous surfaces. The epithelium becomes flattened and disappears, returning to normal on a gluten free diet. It appears that gliadin in the gluten is responsible, as serum antibodies to gliadin are found in the active disease, which reach lower levels during gluten abstinence. But this identification of gliadin does not give a simple answer, as there are no less than 40 protein complexes in gliadin. The exact mechanism of the interaction between dietary gluten and the intestinal mucosa remains to be defined.

Originally it was thought the disease was due to a missing enzyme. But, as Kasarda says 'no-one has been able to demonstrate any enzyme that remains deficient when patients follow a wheat-free diet.' (Cereal Foods World 78 23 (5) pp. 240-4). The most popular theory at present is that it is caused by a primary immunological abnormality. Another scientist, Strumeyer has demonstrated that gliadin has the power to inhibit the activity of human salivary amylase, and could arguably act to depress an already deficient supply of amylase by binding and inactivating amylase secreted into the intestine, thereby interfering with the intestinal hydrolysis of starch. In the absence of amylase, the toxic inhibitor protein would be free to interact with the intestinal mucosa, and cause it damage; whereas excess amylase would remain in normal individuals even after all the inhibitor had become bound to the enzyme (Nutrition Reports Int. 1972 5 pp. 45-52).

Strumeyer's argument appeared to be as relevant to maltose intolerance, including his conclusions on the effect on glucose metabolism, but with the substitution of other inhibitors for gliadin as the depressing factor.

115

I have argued that my family's problem is one of starch digestion, and that we have demonstrated it to our satisfaction on an empirical basis over the years, first with one generation, then the next. One observer has become multiplied at least into three. However biochemistry cannot offer anything more than educated guesses as rationale for our problem, despite the most amazing advances in analytical technique and results in the past decade. There is still too much inconsistency in result. Perhaps when Dr. Archer said I was twenty five years too early for any watertight explanation of my problems, he should have said fifty years.

Take Strumeyer's analysis of gliadin (in gluten) for example. In 1972 he extracted an inhibitor from gliadin that was active against human salivary alpha-amylase enzymes at 100-fold lower concentration than that needed to inhibit pancreatic amylase in pigs (Nutr. Rep. Int. 6 p. 45). However Pace et al 6 years later were unable to detect that any of a number of purified gliadin fractions, including several a, b, and y gliadins, inhibited human salivary or porcine pancreatic alpha amylases (Cereal Chemistry 55 p. 244). Silano points out that gliadin cannot be adequately purified. The preparation used in the above experiments might contain 10% albumin. Therefore, the fact that inhibitors could be extracted from wheat flour, that were commonly considered typical of wheat gliadin, could not be considered proof they were of gliadin nature (p. 158 Enzymes 1987 Am. Assn. of Cereal Chemists ed. Kruger, Lineback, and Stauffer). This one example shows how research is built on a shifting sand. The toxic factor in the wheat might after all not be gliadin, but albumin, or perhaps something else again. Such is the complexity of the life forces of plant and man.

I quote this example in view of the fact that Strumeyer asserted a theory that coeliac disease might be caused by the possibility of amylase inhibitors acting to depress an already deficient alpha-amylase enzyme supply. And it would not be beyond the realms of possibility to allege the same theory in our case.

I should redefine enzymes for those who are not scientists. Enzymes are catalysts, which speed up specific reactions- in the case of alpha-amylase and beta-amylase enzymes the degradation of starch. They exist both in the plant foods we eat, and in ourselves. They interact with each other. The level and balance of this interaction depends on the stage of germination of the plant source. This interaction has been studied even more seriously and extensively in breadmaking than humans, because it governs the quality of the bread.

Cereal alpha-amylase enzymes transform the starch from gelatinised starch (after water is added to flour, and active up to 80 degrees C) into dextrins and oligosaccharides. Beta-amylase enzymes generate quantities of maltose, the major saccharides formed during doughmaking. This maltose is fermented more slowly than glucose.

But you, dear reader, may still find it difficult to understand what maltose is. You will not know it as an old familiar kitchen companion like sucrose in all its forms, whether as the dark sticky treacle, or golden syrup, of my youth, or the sweet white granules of crystalline sugar. You will not know it in its many disguises as glucose syrup, whether in Ovaltine or in the sweets from the corner shop. You will not have gone to your chemist and asked to see the bottle of almost colourless heavy viscous liquid that sells as glucose syrup.

You, dear reader, are more at ease if you can identify the cause of your troubles as something that is visible in the environment such as smog, fumes, dust, or blossoms on the bough; or something that is obvious in your breakfast bowl such as bran or wheatgerm, or on the dinner plate such as fat on the meat, red or green high colour in drinks. You prefer to understand only what you can see. The wheat meal grains in the loaf are positive and conspicuous.

But what of the microscopic forces of nature lurking in the living cells of plants in amounts so small you cannot see them? What of the power of life in the tiny clusters of granules in the wheat, in the larger seed of the potato, a power so concentrated in the thin bran layer of wheat, that if you take away that bran, the starch that is left will not grow another seed. You cannot see these forces of life that surge in the seeds when it is fully grown under the right conditions of heat and wet. And part of that surge is the germination of maltose to degrade the starch reserves of the plant. It provides the very thrust of the energy that courses through our lifeblood, as it does in the plant of its origin.

If you cannot imagine that, then imagine the rising, the leavening, of a bread dough if you can. That is the thrust of the diastatic (turning starch into sugar) element of the enzymes

117

generating maltose fermentation to create the glutenous network, which traps the carbon dioxide of its lift. If the generation of maltose is poor, the dough will not rise as well; for it is maltose that is acted upon by amylase enzymes in the wheat flour to produce more maltose in the active stages of fermentation. The rate of maltose formation is highly important, because this rate governs carbon dioxide production.

Every baker must know what defeats or diminishes this process of maltose generation to make a good loaf. He must be expert in the action either of the natural enzymes within the plant or of the artificial substitutions now commonly used in breadmaking as they can be more reliably controlled than the natural elements of the plant now that large scale bakeries use automated machinery. But, whether the catalysts to starch degradation are one or the other, maltose will be present if the fermentation is not long enough.

It requires at least six hours for maltose to be fermented away, as Dr. Zentner of the Bread Research Institute (C.S.I.R.O.) told me 27 years ago, given that the problem of myself and my family was indeed as I was alleging, that we could not eat wheat starch while it still had the capacity for maltose fermentation. We could eat wheat with attached gluten only in a 'long dough' when the diastiatic activity has died down, or as cornflour, which is devoid of any enzyme or 'diastatic' capacity to ferment maltose from starch.

Now I had never properly understood why Dr. Zentner thought a 'long dough' would work. I had merely found that it did. I had always thought of the original percentage of maltose in the grain as a static amount. I had not imagined this fraction ballooning out to a much greater amount in the process of degradation of the starch, as it does not only in the leavening of bread, but even in the processing necessary to make flour. So, when fate took a hand, providing the opportunity for me to speak to him again only a month ago, I asked him the question that had always plagued me. How can such a small amount of maltose cause so much trouble?

Dr. Zentner's answer was very positive. Maltose is a very powerful catalyst capable of breaking up the dextrins in starch created by alpha-amylase. As this process proceeds, large amounts of maltose are produced which are eventually fermented away. What this relationship between the maltose and the amylases is, no-one yet knows exactly. What is known is that only traces of

118

enzymes are needed to act as catalysts to speed up reactions. Sometimes they are in such minute traces, it is difficult to know they are there.

There is little possibility that my family's problems are not merely due to maltose intolerance, but also to gluten. I have described how I ran a test. I consumed gluten and cornflour as a 'reconstituted' wheat flour for six weeks in breakfast pancakes without any marked reactions. I have recorded how my children and grandchildren can eat bread made on Dr. Zentner's formula of a long dough without any conspicuous symptoms. I have also emphasised that we can produce symptoms merely by eating various products that contain glucose syrup when no gluten is present, the worst reactions being from the high conversion maltose syrups. I have also given details of blind trials, confirming the truth of the latter statement.

I have not ignored the problem inherent in the assertion of maltose intolerance, namely that maltose is produced from other starch resources like corn, and potatoes, which for this reason are used as a source in the manufacture of glucose syrups. This might well have prompted me to insist that gluten was a collateral problem for us to maltose intolerance, as neither of these foodstuffs contain gluten, nor does rice. But clearly such an argument does not stand up.

Therefore I was prompted to look for some other difference between these foods that might explain problems with one, and not with others. There was no facile answer to the enigma, such as the coeliacs had with their gluten. My first thought of course was that the answer lay in the frequency with which certain foods were eaten, as there was no doubt that the effects on us were cumulative. This answer held for corn, but not for potatoes, which we did eat every day.

When I first heard of anti-nutrients in the carbohydrate of raw foodstuffs, I became intrigued with the subject. The same problem existed as with maltose, in that anti-nutrients were widely dispersed through those raw foods. However, an important difference was soon apparent. The levels of these anti-nutrients were dependent on the methods of processing, preparation and cooking. If it transpired the foods we could tolerate easily emerged from the kitchen under different conditions from those that applied to the cereal grains that troubled us, namely, wheat, oats, barley, and rye, then some important explanation might be found. I soon

119

found this research was far more complicated than it would appear to be on the surface.

Then suddenly I found an answer that resolved the complexity. This answer lay in old folk-wisdom about food and the kitchen. I came by the answer when researching the reason why oats must have been a more tolerable food to the Irish with their coeliac propensity in the old days. I found that it had been subject to long preparation, even fermentation, in days gone by. This was true of foods across the world in a'score of different cultures. It was soon clear that we had abandoned many of these practices. A great deal of our food is lightly processed, even raw. If it were true that anti-nutrients would still be present in most of our foodstuffs in such case, and that anti-nutrients could impair starch and protein digestion in various ways, then this fact might be extremely important to anyone supposed to have any problem with starch digestion such as we had with maltose intolerance. The reason for that maltose intolerance was not important. What was important was that if anti-nutrients affected Mr. and Mrs. Average, they would be even more certain to affect us. Had we then managed to eliminate anti-nutrients along with our reduced maltose levels? Had our choice of corn as an ingredient of diet been advantageous because it is almost devoid of alpha-amylase inhibitors?

I spent months hunting down articles on the subject, and backtracking through our diet to see whether this were so. I was amazed to find in a great many cases it was. The flours we tolerated badly such as whole wheat and rye were those where the anti-nutrients were still high. But they had virtually disappeared in the ultra-refined flours we tolerated best, such as wheat and corn starch, or in flours after long fermentation and baking. There was plenty of evidence that water and heat did much to reduce the cumulative effect of anti-nutrients, so that our switch to substituting various tubers wherever possible in our diet became important. Various vegetables and legumes were boiled and steamed. Tubers were often baked. Potatoes were fried. Fruits, including tomatoes, were often brought to the boil.

The conclusion I drew from this intensive re-examination was twofold. The dietetic pattern my mother followed on the whole had given a favourable environment for my impaired glucose tolerance. But I had perforce converted that 'favourable' to an optimum in two respects. I had further eliminated the use of whole white wheat flour, rye or oatmeal in all cakes, biscuits, puddings breakfast foods, or breads, unless fermented for a long time. I had

120

reduced milk consumption, and rejected any recipes such as baked milk puddings which exposed milk to prolonged temperature, or utilised condensed milk, skimmed milk or powder. I do not mention glucose syrup in this context, as it was unknown in household diet at that time.

What I am alleging of course is that maltose intolerance is relative, not absolute. It is not an intolerance to maltose wherever it occurs, but only to maltose under certain conditions. These include grains for reasons not yet fully determined, perhaps the nature of the protein, perhaps the size of the granule, perhaps the types of inhibitors present, perhaps the form in which it is commonly consumed, perhaps because of its predominance in our diet, perhaps because the niacin is bound. There are many 'perhaps', and only scientists in the end can answer these 'perhaps's'.

Our maltose intolerance is relative also insofar as it fluctuates according to the balance, or imbalance, of such maltose with other components of the diet. This becomes particularly obvious when glucose syrups intrude into our diet unwittingly, as they are hard to avoid, being now so ubiquitous throughout household foods. A fair indicator of the enormous level of use is the figure given for the production of D glucose in America alone in 1978, namely some four million tons. The reaction to such glucose syrup may depend on other ingredients consumed at the same time, or the existence of various inhibitors that have not been inactivated.

It is a fascinating subject. I cannot agree with doctors, who are prone to dismiss the question, that my family is very rare. They are thinking I am advancing a medical profile that is one of crisis. I am not. I am describing a profile of twilight health, that may become the future diabetes, or cancer, in middle or late age. I am suggesting this twilight health never attracts attention as due to a single carbohydrate problem, because it is considered a whole spectrum of unrelated problems.

The problem lies not so much with the state of medical research as with the state of biochemical research, where I believe many future medical answers will be found. Some idea of the scope of the problem facing biochemical research are stated in a compendium published by the American Association of Cereal Chemists called 'Enzymes', ed. by Kruger, Lineback, and Stauffer. The series of papers was on the subject of the role of enzymes in cereal technology.

In a chapter on alpha-amylase inhibitors, Silano's words in conclusion exemplify some of the uncertainty of the researcher. 'On the whole, the available data suggests that the cereal and legume alpha-amylase inhibitors in human diets are probably of no nutritional significance for healthy people. Note, however, that all data available refer to short-term testing only. In other words, it is not known whether chronic ingestion of active alpha-amylase inhibitors might excessively stimulate the pancreatic functions to a toxicologically significant extent. The dose-dependent increases in the relative weight of pancreas, observed by Granum and Eskeland (1981) in both rats and chickens after administration of moderate amounts of wheat inhibitors for one to three weeks, deserve additional consideration in relation to this point. They suggest that the amounts of active amylase inhibitors in the diets of patients with impaired proteolysis should be kept as low as possible' (p. 185 'Enzymes').

I put this book down wondering just whether the term 'impaired proteolysis' need necessarily apply to abnormal people, since it could as easily apply to normal people in view of a study which 'demonstrated that high-fibre diets cause a significant decrease in apparent protein digestibility' (Cereal Chemistry 60 (4) 1983 p. 262).

Silano offers an explanation of one variable of our maltose intolerance I had never seen before. He mentions the fact that some alpha-amylase inhibitors may exhibit relative thermal stability, and persist to some extent through baking, since they are found in a considerable number of cooked cereal foodstuffs for human consumption. He adds that 'about 10-20% of the original inhibitory activity towards human salivary alpha-amylase has been found in baked wheat and rye bread (Kneen and Sandstedt 1943) whereas less than 2% of inhibitory activity remained in spaghetti after 15 minutes of boiling (pp. 141-191 'Enzymes'). This finding might be relevant to the fact we found boiled noodles more acceptable than baked wheat biscuits and cakes.

Silano does not express the same caution about the fact these inhibitors may substantially decrease starch availability. He quotes an experiment whereby this occurred when 2.4 to 8% inhibitors were added to diet, a result that did not occur when the inhibitor-loaded starch was autoclaved, or when sucrose was used instead of starch. He also warns of the nutritional danger of several inhibitors active against other proteases, such as subtilin and trypsin. These, he says, may have all the features necessary to

122

make them significant in nutritional terms and theoretically undesirable as food components (p. 191 op. cit.).

Silano lists some of the substances that may reduce the activity of one or more alpha-amylases of different origins. I found the list both surprising and puzzling. Some are less surprising than others, e.g. aspirin, drugs like tetracycline and salicylic acid. Some are interesting, like the use of surfactants (that coat the surface of granules). Some are more obscure, like low-molecular weight compounds, or macromolecules, either produced by microorganisms or occuring naturally in plants. Some are frankly puzzling, like 'end products of alpha-amylase action on starch'. But the most astonishing of all in my book was the declaration that maltose, maltotriose, maltotetraose, and some of their reduced analogs also exhibit alpha-amylase inhibiting activity, since they can be attracted to a substrate that looks similar. How I longed to know what substrates, and the effect this kidnapping of any of the maltose triumvirate would have, and regretted my basic ignorance of science.

And yet, a few further pages along, one reads what appears to be the opposite- that 'under inhibition assay conditions, maltose stops some of the inhibition of insect, avian and human amylase.' Silano details experiments with maltose added to a preincubated solution of enzyme and inhibitor performed by others. He adds that maltose did not reverse the reaction between the rye inhibitor and human salivary alpha-amylase when added after complex formation, but it did reduce the extent of complex formation when added at the same time as the inhibitor (p. 176 op. cit.).

All very heady stuff, in which one fact stood out above all others. Interaction was all important, and the sequence in which dietary components were added governed the extent of the inhibition. Not a balanced diet, but the balance of diet. I longed for a true knowledge of science to understand it all. I felt despair, and total agreement with Professor Fraser when he said I had reached the stage when I must leave explanations to the scientists, to men whose work Stauffer says early in the book is still full of inconsistencies and disagreements, to researchers who have not even standardised their nomenclature in some areas of debate, let alone resolved all problems of analytical method. In a separate publication of the American Association of Cereal Chemists, 'Cereal Polysaccharides in Technology and Nutrition', Kruger says further 'the precise nature of the products formed from the

123

degradation of wheat starch granules is still unknown and more research is needed in this area in the future' (p. 31).

Change is the name of the game. For example, Dr. Brand of the Nutrition Department of the University of Sydney handed me a sheet only this week on the very point I have been discussing- namely, the action of alpha-amylase enzymes on starch. Three different a-glucosidases, attached to the limiting membrane of the microvilli which line the small intestinal mucosa, are capable of hydrolysing maltose, maltotriose and a-dextrins to free glucose. Until now, they have always been called maltases. But it has been found that maltose is not the most important physiological substrate for two of these enzymes. Therefore they are no longer called maltases, but distinguished as glucoamylase, a-dextrinase, and sucrase. A-dextrins are thought to be the most physiologically significant substrate of the former two, and actions on maltose and maltotriose, as well as sucrose, in the case of the latter. This kind of change in definition, and analysis, does not seem to invalidate any of my conclusions. Indeed it appears to offer some explanation why in past years I had found I maintained stability in the children by reducing the degree to which sucrose was associated with starch degradation involving these dextrins and maltose. In other words, I watched carefully how and where they were associated together. For example, a domestic cake or biscuit was preferable to high-conversion syrups or ice-cream, and choices could be made at birthday parties in those terms.

As I have emphasised before, any attempt to explain this world of the enzymes that coordinate the sequence of changes in development and germination is difficult because their dynamics are invisible. The best way for a layman to comprehend it is through the visible miracle of leavening of bread, through watching bread rise as the yeast works on the starch to ferment the bread, we have an insight into digestion. However in the case of the latter we have no gauge to see what goes wrong, no high or low loaf. We cannot judge by eye or feel what is happening in the body. If the amylase enzymes are too low, and the starch is not being adequately degraded, this can only be supposed by differential diagnosis.

People of different cultures have developed many aids to digestion over the centuries. Milk of magnesia for stomach upset. Papain from pawpaw and pineapple, yeast and yoghurt for effective protease and bacterial action. Bicarbonate of soda for release of bound niacin. Salt for other cooking values. Potatoes or

124

taro for baby food. Arrowroot and groats for sickly children. Indeed, oats interestingly were never considered acceptable as food outside Germany or Britain except for the relief of stomach discomfort and invalids.

The failure of oats to spread through Europe, or anywhere else, as a staple of diet until very recent times is interesting in view of the fact we now know that the protein of oats is higher in quantity, and 15-20% better than other cereals in quality, and that the water soluble fatty acids are better for health than those in wheat.

But what this small book is concerned with ultimately is not to advocate the diet of other cultures, even my own, but only the diet that I was obliged to adopt. This was a very modified form of my grandmother's diet. This must be the last word in this book, because it is the only word I can assert positively as a truth- not a universal truth, but a truth for myself and certain members of my family. Our maltose intolerance diet is valid for us, no more.

The general principles are as follows-

EXCLUSIONS

1. No wheat unless fermented at least six hours.
2. No oats or barley unless soaked, slow boiled a long time. No beer.
3. No rye, unless well fermented. (Rye breads are mainly wheat).
4. No milk if skimmed, condensed, boiled, superheated, 'longlife', yoghurt or buttermilk from skimmed milk. No cottage cheese.
5. No glucose syrup, maltose "sugar" syrup, malto-dextrins, glucose.
6. No honey, grapes, or wine.
7. No quantity of fruit juice, particularly reconstituted juice, except for pineapple juice.
8. No daily quantity of raw salad vegetables and fruit.
9. No raw or lightly roasted nuts.
10. No lightly processed soya flour except in small quantities.
11. No cereal bran of any kind, or wheat germ. No 'fibre'. No 'brown' rice.
12. No sugars of any kind without fats and protein.
13. No icecreams unless made with whole milk, cream and sucrose.
14. No sucrose, when split into fructose/glucose by acid fruits in jams, pies, cordials etc.
15. No corn chips, or cornflakes with added malto-dextrins.

INCLUSIONS

1. Rice of any variety, ground rice, and rice flour.
2. Corn of any variety, whole, flour, tortillas, popcorn etc. Not daily.
3. Potatoes of any variety, whether as chips, dumplings, or vegetables.
4. Tubers such as carrots, parsnips, etc., boiled, baked or casseroled. Or, in the case of carrots, in carrot cakes.
5. Sweet potatoes in any form.
6. Ultra-refined starches from any source. Wheat or maize cornflour. Tapioca flour. Arrowroot. Taro flour. Potato flour. Besant flour.
7. Sucrose whether table sugar, white or brown, treacle, golden syrup.
8. Milk in small quantities, but not one glass at a time. Butter, cream, cream cheese, cheese, cream buttermilk, sour cream.
9. Beans of any kind, if well cooked at high temperatures.
10. Fruit of any kind, especially coconuts, bananas and pineapple, and fruit that is neither too unripe nor too ripe. In moderate quantities, and preferably with a meal.
11. Any sources of protein other than cereals. Eggs, and red meat, are particularly beneficial for complete protein, iron, trace elements.
12. Foods that are well cooked at temperatures above 100 degrees, as in steaming and baking.
13. Vegetables, rice, beans and other foods well soaked in lukewarm water before cooking. Potatoes with added salt.
14. Sucrose, when in its original form, and not inverted.

I take leave of this book at this point with relief. Three rewrites to try to make a simple statement have left me in a state of mental exhaustion as if I had written a doctorate thesis. Yet there can be no end to the story. More work lies beyond.

Already while this finale is being written, Dr. Zentner rang me to say he had just heard a radio program on melanoidinins as a cause of cataracts in the eye. These are produced in the Maillard browning reaction of a baked loaf, whereby the combination of sugars with certain amino acids forms the crust. Would I carry out just one more test? My first reaction was oh no, not another experiment which will give me bloodshot eyes and last for days affecting my concentration. Not a revival of the old bread-making techniques I had practised for years.

I asked what the test would be. He said it would be to make a bread dough, to let it prove for just one hour, then divide it in half, and cook one half in the microwave, and the other in the ordinary oven. This would test whether the lack of a brown crust in the microwave loaf would make the bread any more acceptable to my metabolism.

Fortunately, I had the book on cereal technology at my elbow with a discourse on this very reaction, the bakers' concern being to keep it at an acceptable level so the outside crust of a given loaf would not be too solid and heavy. One cause of this Maillard reaction, it seems, is what is known in the trade as a 'green' loaf from an excess of alpha-amylase in the wheat flour itself, or some analagous cause.

I must admit I quailed at the very thought. Imagine tracking back through all my thought processes to relate the thought of these new little irritants to any of our past observations. All very well for a computer which can activate its tireless chips, and riffle through its files to throw answers up on a screen. My brain is tired. My files have already been cast down. I throw the gauntlet now to others, hoping they will throw it back to me with the answer that has not yet been thrown up on my screen, before my grandchildren have reached what used to be known as their full estate. With this wish, I say farewell, dear reader, even as I leave the house to drive up to the baker to beg enough high gluten flour to make those loaves for Dr. Zentner. Your last glimpse of me will be slaving away over that dough in the heat of my kitchen.

Oh yes, a tome on bread-making over 500 years at my side, extracting a list of unprocurable items to revive the lost art of ancient baking. Earthenware pots, glazed inside and not outside. Terracotta tiles for the oven instead of trays. Flower pots to invert over the bread. Cheesecloth for pegtub cold water eighteen-hour doughs.

Crinkle bread my baker's grandfather used to make in Denmark- the best bread in the world he said today. So if you wander in and find the dough rising in the shower recess while I have my shower, or in the bathtub, or baking in a flowerpot in the oven, or rising in a Chinese soup cauldron, please do not think I have lost my marbles. I have it on the best authority that way lies bread to win your heart.

FINIS- OCTOBER 17, 1989

A LOW MALTOSE/GLUCOSE/LACTOSE DIET.

BASIC INGREDIENTS

FLOURS	Starches up to 90% (alone or together)	Cornflour - maize or wheat potato flour rice flour tapioca maize polenta taro(if available) arrowroot
	high protein flour (10%)	soya flour
FATS	low lactose	butter cream sour cream cheese(except cottage cheese) lard (excellent for pastries)
LIQUIDS	Low-lactose (for mineral supplement)	whole milk only juices in moderation blackcurrant and pineapple
SWEETENER	sucrose	tinned fruit in natural juices jam (but not with added glucose)
RAISING AGENT	as normal, but increased slightly.	baking powder cream of tartar/bicarb soda or GDL/bicarb soda 2/1 2 teaspoons per cup or 4oz

128

BASIC COOKING FOR NON-WHEAT FLOURS.

(1) Soya flour should be creamed with shortening, and blended with liquids if there is residual fat in the flour (some is defatted). Do not mix with dry flour.

(2) The mixture should not be too thick, as the flours used respond in a slightly different way to wheat flour.

(3) The baking temperature should be reduced 25 degrees below the temperature specified to prevent excess browning.

(4) Cakes and biscuits are best left to cool for a time on racks or in tins, before lifting or turning out, due to the finer texture of the product.

(5) Milk should be whole milk, not dry milk and cooked slowly without bringing to the boil.

(6) Eggs and milk are best at room temperature.

(7) Egg white, guar gum, or glyceryl monostereate can help to give binding qualities in non-wheat mixtures for pastries and pieshells.

(8) More raising agent should be used than with normal wheat flour.

(9) The best fat, particularly for sponges is either fat, or 2 parts of butter for 1 of lard.

(10) The best fat for making pastry with fine flour, particularly rice pastry, is lard.

BASIC RECIPES

These recipes presume the flours used are combinations of flours as listed in the chapter on alternative flours.
1) The cakes, scones and biscuits are indistinguishable from normal with experience.
2) The pancakes and pizzas are different from normal in the absence of gluten (protein), which gives wheat flour its unique leavening properties. But they are quite acceptable to children.
3) The pieshells give scope for more inventive alternatives.
4) Desserts provide the greatest range of normal alternatives as many traditional recipes use alternative starches.

1. BISCUITS

PEANUT WAFERS

8 oz chopped peanuts	Blend all ingredients.
2 eggs	Roll dough to 1/2 thickness.
4 oz white sugar	Cut into strips 4x1 inches.
1/2 teaspoon salt	Bake on a well-greased tray
1 oz butter	for twenty minutes.
1 tablespoon milk	
8 oz flour (wheat substitute)	

FRENCH FLORENTINES

4 oz butter	Melt butter and sugar together.
4 oz castor sugar	Stir in other ingredients except
4 oz chopped almonds	chocolate, sliced almonds.
3 oz plain chocolate	Add beaten egg.
1 oz sliced almonds	Spoon small heaps of mixture on
2 oz candied peel	greased tray.
2 oz chopped walnuts	Press almond strips on top.
1 oz glace cherries	Bake 20-25 minutes at 350 degrees.
	Cool before inverting on wire rack.
	Coat bottoms with melted
	chocolate.

ALMOND MERINGUES

2 egg whites	Beat eggs until stiff.
4 oz castor sugar	Gradually fold in 3 ozs of
Vanilla	chopped nut brittle and vanilla.
Nut brittle	Fold in balance of sugar.
1 oz silvered almonds	Spoon on tray. Sprinkle almonds.
	Bake 25 minutes in a slow oven.
	(Nut Brittle—Coat 8 oz roasted
	almonds with sugar melted to a
	thin syrup, and spread to cool).

RICE BISCUITS.

4 oz ground rice	Cream butter and sugar.
1 egg	Add vanilla, then lemon juice.
4 oz cornflour	Blend a small portion of the flour.
1 teaspoon baking powder	Beat egg well in.
4 oz castor sugar	Add the rest of the flour.
3 oz butter	Form the mixture into small balls.
1 teaspoon lemon juice	Place on tray and flatten.
1/2 teaspoon vanilla.	Garnish with almond sliver.
1/4 teaspoon salt	Bake at 350 (180) degs 15-20
	minutes.

PITCARTHLY BANNOCK

1/2 cup butter	Cream butter and sugar.
1/4 cup sugar	Beat in flour, almonds and peel
1/4 cup flour	Flatten a square sheet 5 mm thick.
1/4 cup rice flour	Chill one hour.
1/2 cup ground almonds	Crimp edges. Mark off rectangles.
1/3 cup ground lemon peel	Bake 300 (150) degs one hour.

SHORTBREAD BISCUITS

4 oz butter
1/4 cup icing sugar
1/4 cup plain flour
1 cup cornflour
1/2 teaspoon baking powder.
Glace cherries

Preheat oven 375 (190) degs
Beat butter and sugar to a cream.
Sift flours and baking powder.
Spoon teaspoons of mix on tray.
Top each with a glace cherry.
Bake 350 (180) 20 Minutes. Cool on tray.

DATE COOKIES

1 egg
6 tablespoons sugar
3/4 cup chopped dates
1 teaspoon vanilla
1+1/2 cups rice bubbles
3/4 cup coconut

Stir sugar and dates in beaten egg.
Heat in pan until dates are pasty.
Stir in vanilla and cereal.
Mould small balls.
Roll in coconut. Cool until firm.

CORNFLAKE NUT DAINTIES

Whites of 2 eggs
3/4 cup of sugar
2/3 cup of coconut
4 cups cornflakes
1/2 teaspoon salt
vanilla
2 tablespoons butter

Beat whites.
Add sugar and salt.
Beat well again.
Stir in other ingredients.
Add melted butter.
Spoon onto greased tray.
Bake 300 (150) degs 20 minutes.

SWEET POTATO BISCUITS

2 cups flour
4 teaspoons baking powder
1 teaspoon salt
1/4 cup sugar
2 cups cooked sweet potatoes
1/2 cup butter
3/4 cup milk or cream

Preheat oven to 425 (200) degs.
Sift dry ingredients.
Blend sweet potatoes and butter.
Add milk to make a soft dough.
Knead on floured board till smooth.
Roll out to 1/2 inch thickness.
Cut rounds with biscuit cutter.
Bake rounds 10-15 minutes.

SWEET POTATO BALLS

2 cups cooked sweet potato
1 large ripe banana
1+1/2 tablespoons melted butter
1 1egg yolk
1+1/2 teaspoons salt
1/4 cup cream, nutmeg, or ginger
1 egg white

Blend mashed. banana/sweet
potato.
Blend with butter, egg, salt, milk,
flavouring.
Fold in beaten egg white.
Spoon in mounds on greased tray.
Bake 500 (250) degrees 12 minutes.

CHOCOLATE CRACKLES.

1/2 cup copha butter
3 tablespoons cocoa
1/2 lb icing sugar
5 cups rice bubbles

Melt copha butter.
Add cocoa and icing sugar.
Pour in rice bubbles.
Stir until well coated.
Spoon into paper cups and cool.

LOVE BALLS.

Weight of three eggs in
-butter
-sugar
-flour
(add baking powder at
2 teaspoons per cup)

Cream butter and sugar.
Stir in eggs.
Blend in flour to a very stiff mix.
If not stiff enough, add flour and
cornflour in turn.
Shape into small balls.
Bake 400 (200) degrees 15 minutes.

133

CORNFLAKE BISCUITS.

1 cup flour	Sift flour and baking powder.
2 teaspoons baking powder	Add coconut, cornflakes and sugar.
1 cup coconut	Pour over melted butter.
1 cup cornflakes	Press into flat biscuit tin.
1/2 cup brown sugar	Mix juice and icing sugar.
5/8 lb butter	Pour over while hot.
Juice of 1 lemon	Cut into squares while cooling.
Icing sugar as required	

PAVLOVA BISCUITS

2 egg whites	Beat egg whites stiffly.
4 oz sugar	Fold in sugar, then other items.
1 oz cornflour	Spoon in small mounds on tray.
1 dessertspoon chocolate	Bake 250 (150) degs 45 minutes.
2 oz chopped nuts	

BRANDY SNAPS

1/3 cup treacle	Melt sugar, treacle, butter over a
1/2 cup brown sugar	low heat.
3 oz butter	Add flour, flavourings and brandy.
1/4 teaspoon ground ginger	Roll into 3/4 inch balls.
1/2 teaspoon cinnamon	Bake 300 (160) 12 minutes.
1/2 teaspoon lemon/orange rind	Leave a minute or so.
2 teaspoons brandy	Remove with spatula.
1 cup flour	Roll over spoon handle.

SCOTCH SHORTBREAD

1 cup sugar
6 oz butter
2 eggs
1/4 cup sour cream
2 cups flour
4 teaspoons baking powder

Cream butter and sugar.
Add other ingredients.
Chill dough several hours until
easy to handle.
Press dough into trays.
Bake 375 (18) 20 minutes.

RICH ROCK CAKES

1/2 cup sugar
1+1/2 cups flour
3 teaspoons baking powder
1 cup sultanas
1/2 cup mixed peel
1 cup seeded raisins
1 egg
4 oz butter
1 teaspoon cinnamon
1 teaspoon ground ginger
1 teaspoon mixed spice

Cream butter and sugar.
Beat in egg.
Sift flour/baking powder.
Add flour/fruit in turn.
Stir well.
Spoon small pieces on tray.
Bake 400 (200) 20 minutes.

MACAROONS

4 oz castor sugar
2 oz ground almonds
1 teaspoon ground rice
White 1 large egg
1 teaspoon water

Mix dry ingredients.
Stir in egg white.
Add water. Beat well.
Drop spoonsfuls on tray.
Bake at 300 (150) 15 mins.

2. CAKES

CHOCOLATE SANDWICH CAKE

6 oz flour
3 teaspoons baking powder
2 oz cooking chocolate
(or 4 tablespoons cocoa)
1/2 teaspoon salt
1/3 cup mashed potato
4 oz butter
4 tablespoons milk
2 eggs

Cream potato, butter, sugar.
Add melted chocolate or cocoa.
Add beaten eggs alternately with
flour and salt.
Mix in milk.
Add mixture to two 8" tins.
Bake 400 (200) degrees 25-30 mins.
Join with filling of choice.

COCONUT CAKE

1/2 cup butter
3/4 oz sugar
2 eggs separated
1+1/2 cups potato flour
1/2 teaspoon baking powder
3 tablespoons jam

Cream butter and sugar.
Beat in egg yolks, then potato flour
and baking powder.
Pour into a lamington tin.
Bake 300 (150) 20 minutes.
Melt jam in water, add to
beaten whites, sugar, coconut.
Top and bake 15 minutes.

POTATO FRUIT BUN

1/2 cup cold mashed potato
1/2 cup castor sugar
1/2 cup sultanas
1/2 cup currants
1 egg
1 oz melted butter
1/4 cup milk
1/2 teaspoon vanilla
1 cup flour
2 teaspoons baking powder
Lemon juice

Mix sugar, potato, sultanas and
currants with the sifted flour.
Add beaten egg, melted butter, milk
and vanilla until a dough.
Place in an 8" tin.
Bake 300 (180) for 30 minutes.
Cool on a wire rack.
Spread thin lemon icing on top.
(Icing—one dessertspoonful
lemon juice in 1/2 cup icing sugar.)

BANANA CAKE

8 oz flour
1 teaspoon bicarbonate of soda
3-4 ripe bananas
2 eggs
4 oz butter
4 oz sugar
1 oz lemon rind

Cream sugar and butter.
Add well-beaten egg, flour and
mashed bananas.
Dissolve bicarb. soda in milk.
Divide mix in sandwich tins.
Bake 375 (190) for one hour.
Fill with lemon icing.

SPONGE CAKE

3 eggs separated
pinch salt
1/4 teaspoon vanilla
1/2 cup castor sugar
2/3 cup corn flour
1 tablespoon flour
1 teaspoon baking powder

Pre-heat oven 375 (190) degs.
Add salt to egg whites.
Beat until soft peaks form.
Add sugar until stiff.
Blend in egg yolks and vanilla.
Sift flours and baking powder.
Fold in egg mixture with a wooden
spoon or spatula.
Bake 20 minutes in two tins.

RICE OR POTATO FLOUR SPONGE CAKE

3 cups rice or potato flour
1/2 cup sugar
8 egg yolks
9 egg whites

Sift flour 3 times with sugar.
Stir yolks into flour mixture.
Fold whites gently in.
Pour into cake tin.
Bake 350 (180) 55 minutes.
Do not cut with a knife.

CONTINENTAL RICE CAKE

8 oz ready-cooked rice
3 eggs (separated)
1 tablespoon cornflour
2 ozs castor sugar
1/2 cup cornflake crumbs
1/2 cup sour cream
grated rind of one lemon

Beat sugar into the whites.
Fold milk, beaten yolk, rice,
cornflour and rind into whites.
Toss crumbs into cake tin.
Pre-heat oven to 425 (220) degs.
Cook at 300 (150) 30 mins.
Serve hot or cold, topped with
cinnamon, jam or sauces.

RICE MUFFINS (1)

8 oz flour
4 teaspoons baking powder
pinch salt
2 oz cold boiled rice
1 oz melted fat
1 egg
1/4 pint milk

Combine flour, baking powder, salt
with the rice.
Add cooled fat, eggs and milk.
Blend well with flour.
Bake 400 (200) until firm and
brown.

FOR SAVOURY MUFFINS:

seasoning
3 oz grated cheese
pepper
mustard

FOR SWEET MUFFINS:

2 oz sugar.
2 oz dried fruit

RICE MUFFINS (2)

1 cup rice flour
2 teaspoons baking powder
1/2 teaspoon salt
1 cup milk
1 oz butter, jam or
marmalade
raisins

Mix flour, salt, baking powder and
sugar together.
Melt butter, and cool slightly.
Add to beaten egg and milk.
Blend flour with egg mixture.
Add jam/marmalade/raisins.
Bake 400 (200) 12-15 minutes.

ONE STOP CAKE

2 eggs	Beat eggs and sugar together.
3/4 cup sugar	Sift flour and baking powder.
2 cups flour	Add to egg mixture.
4 teaspoons baking powder	Stir in milk and butter.
3/4 cup milk	Add flavourings of choice.
1/4 lb melted butter	Bake 375 (180) 30 minutes.

CHOCOLATE CAKE

6 oz butter	Cream butter and sugar until light.
9 oz castor sugar	Add egg yolks. Beat well.
6 eggs separated	Add breadcrumbs.
3 oz breadcrumbs	Melt chocolate in hot water.
4 oz milk chocolate	Add mix to ground almonds.
5 oz bitter chocolate	Beat stiff whites into mix.
5+1/2 ground almonds	Bake 375 (180) for 1 hour.
2 tablespoons water	

DOUBLE-DELIGHT CHOCOLATE CAKE

6 ozs cream cheese	Cream cheese, half butter,
1 cup butter	and flavours until fluffy.
1/2 teaspoon vanilla	Blend in half icing sugar.
1/2 teaspoon peppermint	Add hot water alternately
6 cups sifted icing sugar	with the balance of the icing sugar.
1/4 cup hot water	Blend in melted chocolate.
4 ozs melted chocolate	Half is for frosting,half for filling.
2+1/4 cups sifted flour	Blend rest with half butter
2 teaspoons baking powder	the eggs one at a time.
1 teaspoon salt	Add sifted flour and milk in turn.
3 eggs	Pour into two pans.
3/4 cup milk	Bake 350 (160) 35 minutes.

3. *FLAT GRIDDLE CAKES*

Notes on pancakes.
    (a) Mix liquid into dry ingredients with quick strokes.
    (b) Ignore lumps.
    (c) Allow to rest, covered, 3 to 6 hours before cooking.
    (d) Do not grease if recipe has ample butter.
    (e) The pan is ready when cold water drops bounce on pan.

RICE GRIDDLE CAKES

1 1/4 cups flour	Mix flour, salt, baking powder.
1/2 teaspoon salt	Stir in milk.
2 teaspoons baking powder	Add rice, butter and egg.
1+1/4 cups milk	Drop tablespoons of the mixture on
1+1/4 cups cooked rice	hot oiled pan.
1+1/2 tablespoons melted butter	Serve with butter and syrup.
1 beaten egg	

LACY CORN BREAD

1 cup yellow corn meal	Mix corn meal, flour, salt and
1/2 cup flour	baking powder in a bowl.
2 teaspoons baking powder	Mix with water to a thin batter.
1/2 teaspoon salt	Pour into oil when almost smoking.
1+1/2 cups water	Turn when the top is lacy, and the
peanut oil	bottom brown.
	Drain on paper towels.
	Thin batter if too thick.

FADGE

5 medium boiled potatoes	Mash 2 tablespoons butter into the
4 tablespoons flour	hot potatoes.
1/2 cup grated cheddar cheese	Mix flour well in.
1/2 teaspoon dry mustard	Blend cheese and flavourings.
4 tablespoons butter	Roll out to 1/2 inch thickness.
1 teaspoon salt	Cut into shapes and triangles.
1/2 teaspoon pepper	Brush on melted butter.
1 tablespoon chopped chives	Fry 5 mins each side in pan, or bake
	350 (190) 30 mins.

4. BREADS

VIVIAN'S CORN BREAD

2 cups yellow corn meal	Pre-heat oven to 400 (200).
1 cup flour	Sift corn meal, baking powder, and
1 tablespoon baking powder	flour.
2 lightly beaten eggs	Add eggs, salt, sugar, butter and
1 teaspoon salt	milk.
1 cup milk	Bake in 9 inch square pan.
3 tablespoons butter	Leave 20-25 minutes, or until firm in
	the centre.

BANANA BREAD

1/2 cup butter	Cream butter and sugar.
3/4 cup sugar	Add well beaten eggs.
2 eggs	Stir in soda, and bananas.
2 ripe bananas	Then the whole with flour.
2 teaspoons bicarbonate soda	Bake 350 (180) for 50 minutes.
2 cups flour	

PUMPKIN BREAD

1+1/4 cups sugar	Pre-heat oven to 350 (180).
1/3 cup butter	Cream butter and sugar.
2 eggs	Beat in eggs, one at a time.
1 cup mashed pumpkin	Stir in pumpkin.
1+1/4 cups flour	Sift dry ingredients together.
1/4 teaspoonful baking powder	Add alternately with water.
1/4 teaspoon ground cloves	Stir in nuts.
1/2 teaspoon cinnamon	Spoon batter into loaf tin.
3/4 teaspoon salt	Bake for 30 minutes.
1/2 cup chopped nuts	
1/3 cup water	

5. DESSERTS

DATE BUTTERSCOTCH PUDDING

2 oz sago	Cover sago with water.
1 pint water	Stir and leave to settle.
vanilla	Pour off water.
2 oz brown sugar	Stir in boiling liquid 15 minutes.
pinch salt	Add sugar, dates and spice.
1/2 cup chopped dates	Serve hot or cold.
1 oz butter	
1/2 teaspoon mixed spice	

RICE SOUFFLE

1 cup rice	Combine rice with cream.
1+1/3 cups light cream	Cook slowly until creamy.
3 egg yolks	Blend yolks 1/4 cup sugar.
1/2 cup sugar	Add raisins softened with water
1/2 cup raisins	and stir well in.
1 teaspoon vanilla	Mix in flavourings.
1 tablespoon lemon rind	Layer the mixture in pie dish with
Whip egg whites with	jam if desired.
1+1/4 cups of sugar.	Arrange on top.
3 stiffly beaten egg whites	Bake 350 (175) 20 minutes.
2 tablespoons butter	Pour and fire warm brandy.
1/2 cup raspberry or other jam	
1 small glass brandy	

BANANA TRIFLE

6 large ripe bananas
3 tablespoons apricot jam
1 tablespoon gelatine
1/4 pint boiling water
3 level tablespoons sugar
6 tablespoons lemon juice
30 small macaroons
1/2 pint custard
1/2 pint whipped cream
2 oz slivered almonds

Mash to a pulp with jam.
Dissolve gelatine first in cold, then boiling water.
Add sugar, sherry, lemon.
Lay macaroons dowsed in sherry on base of bowl.
Add banana jelly, custard, and a layer of macaroons.
Repeat until finished.
Cover with cream.
Garnish with almonds.

TAPIOCA PUDDING

2 cups water
3 tablespoons tapioca
1/2 cup sugar
1/4 teaspoon salt
2 tablespoons lemon juice
2 cups crushed pineapple
pulped apricot
crushed berries

Combine tapioca, sugar, salt with twc cups of boiling water in top of double boiler.
Stir at the boil for 5 minutes.
Remove from heat.
Cool a few minutes.
Blend in fruit of choice.
Serve with cold cream.

SAGO MOULD

2 oz sago
3/4 pint water or fruit juice
pinch salt
juice and rind of a lemon
1 tablespoon treacle
1 tablespoon brown sugar
1 tablespoon butter
(mixed spice if desired).

Soak sago and pour water off.
Add salt to water.
Bring to boil. Add sago.
Stir 15 minutes until clear.
Remove from the fire.
Add lemon, treacle and sugar.
Stir in butter.
Pour in mould to set.
(If adding one or two eggs, use less sago. 1/2 oz or less for one egg. 1 oz for two.

SAGO PLUM PUDDING

2 tablespoons sago
3/4 cup milk
1/4 cup brandy or sherry
2 oz butter
1/2 cup sugar
1 teaspoon bicarb. soda
pinch salt
1 cup crumbs (any kind)
1 cup mixed fruits
2 teaspoons grated lemon rind
1/2 teaspoon mixed spice
1/2 teaspoon ground ginger

Cook sago until transparent.
Add sugar, salt, flavour.
Stir in butter.
Prepare meringue separately.
Beat whites stiff with salt.
Pour in steamer with tight lid.
Steam for two hours.
Add cream or brandy sauce.

DATE PUDDING

3 oz stoned dates
3 oz breadcrumbs
3 ozs flour
3 ozs suet or lard
1 teaspoon cinnamon
1 teaspoon bicarbonate soda
milk as needed

Mix dry ingredients.
If lard used, blend in.
Moisten with milk.
Steam in greased mould.
Microwave (1/2 hour).
Serve with sweet sauce.

RAILWAY PUDDING

4 ozs flour
2 teaspoons baking powder
2 oz sugar
1 1/2 ozs butter
1 egg
1 tablespoon chopped sultanas
2 tablespoons cold milk
grated rind of one lemon

Mix sugar with flour.
Melt butter slightly.
Add to flour.
Add rind and sultanas.
Beat egg. Add milk.
Stir in flour.
Pour in shallow pie dish.
Bake 375 (180) 40 minutes.

144

ORANGE PUDDING

Twice the weight of 2 eggs in
-butter
-flour
2 teaspoons baking powder
1 orange
Sauce-
juice of 1 orange
1/2 pint water
1 oz butter
1/2 oz cornflour
1 tablespoon sugar and brandy

Cream butter and sugar.
Add eggs. Beat well.
Add rind and juice of orange.
Bake microwave 30 minutes.
Melt butter. Add flour.
Stir constantly, while adding
orange juice and water.
Cook gently 5 minutes at boil.
Add sugar and liquor.

6. PIES
SAVOURY PUMPKIN PIE

16 oz pumpkin
4 oz cooked rice
1 small onion
3 tablespoons parsley
1 cup grated tasty cheese
salt and pepper
3 eggs
3 tablespoons milk

Make pastry shell first.
Mix all ingredients together.
Spread evenly over the pastry.
Beat eggs and milk together.
Spread over the pastry.
Glaze with a beaten egg yolk.
Pierce pastry here and there.
Bake 350 (180) for 3/4 hour.

SWEET PUMPKIN PIE

6 oz cooked pumpkin
1 cup cream or 500 grms
cream cheese
6 tablespoons brown sugar
1/2 teaspoon salt
1/2 teaspoon cinnamon
1/2 teaspoon nutmeg
1 teaspoon ginger
pinch of cloves
4 slightly beaten eggs
2 tablespoons rum or brandy
currants and sultanas

Cook pumpkin in double boiler, or
microwave.
Do not boil.
Mash. Add other ingredients.
Cool slightly. Add vanilla, brandy
or rum.
Add to baked pie shell.
Bake at 350 (180) till set.

PAVLOVA

3 egg whites
6 oz castor sugar
cornflour.
vanilla
1/2 teaspoon vinegar
1/2 teaspoon vanilla
1/2 teaspoon cornflour

Beat egg whites until stiff, adding sugar.
Fold in vanilla, vinegar and
Spread mixture in 8 inch circle shell.
Bake 250 (175) 4-5 hours.
Fill with whipped cream, or lemon cheese.
Garnish with cherries, berries.

DE LUXE CHEESE CAKE

2 cups cornflake crumbs
6 tablespoons butter
2 eggs
3/4 lb soft cream cheese
1/2 cup sugar
1 teaspoon lemon juice
or vanilla
1/2 teaspoon salt
1+1/2 cups sour cream
2 tablespoons sugar
1/2 teaspoon vanilla
1/8 teaspoon salt

Melt butter. Pour over crumbs.
Mix well. Chill in pie dish, or bake at 300 (150) degrees.
Blend eggs, cream cheese, sugar, salt and flavour.
Bake 375 (180) 30 minutes.
Dust with cinnamon.
Mix cream sugar and flavours.
Pour over the cake.
Bake 5 minutes to glaze.
Refrigerate 6-12 hours.

OTHER FORMS OF CRUST

Chill well or bake at low temperatures.

(a) Any biscuit or cake crumbs.
   Add icing sugar if plain only, butter, and flavour if needed.
(b) Any cereal crumb, crushed or ground.
   Fill with firm (such as cheesecake or gelatin) fillings.
(c) Cornflour, or rice flour, pastry made with lard to consistency.
   Add iced water. Chill before rolling out.
(d) Potatoes. Cooked mashed potatoes mixed with 1/4 the amount of flour and 1 tablespoon melted butter and salt. Rolled out like pastry.

BREAD, THE STAFF OF LIFE (SOMETIMES)

Throughout this book I have emphasised that my family can only eat wheat as a long-time bread, in other words, a bread baked after the dough has been left to ferment for at least six hours, preferably longer, using only old-fangled ingredients.

This was the kind of bread I was obliged to make for my children throughout the years when they were growing up, because it was no longer made in bakehouses. This was also the kind of bread made universally in the old days, when doughs were given much longer and slower fermentation than today's high speed doughs, based on a few minutes of intensive mechanical agitation in special high speed mixers.

As Elisabeth David says in her book, "Bread and Yeast Cookery" "the true essence of good bread lies in the slow ferment and unhurried ripening of the dough" (p.100). This gives the 'bread-flavour to bread'.

Long-time bread, you may think lightly enough, why, that should be easy. Take a bread recipe for a 2 hour dough. Multiply by 3 or 5, depending on whether you plan a six hour dough, or a 10 hour overnight dough. Put the flour, yeast, salt and water together, and, hey presto, you have your bread. But, hey presto, you do not, as I have found to my cost.

Bread dough can be a fickle, treacherous creature. It may rise remorselessly and bloom out of its container if it is not captured, punched down, and kneaded once more. Or it may sulk, and remain a leaden, grudging lump in the basin. At all times it will involve you in a state of war, not friendship. Why? I never knew why until this week when I set pen to paper. Or should I say set hand to the word processor key board. I had religiously taken the amount of yeast specified on the packet, whether the yeast was fine or coarse granules. I had weighed out the amount prescribed in the recipe books. But none of them, not even the holy writ of Rombauer's " The Joy of Cooking", said a word of warning that long doughs were different. One simply cannot adapt those recipes by the same rule of thumb as for cakes, and batters. Not one of them in fact mentioned long-time doughs at all, even though they were the staple of every mother's kitchen two centuries ago. Such is change. We have moved into the age of hurry-up, and cookbooks cater for speed.

147

What was the word of warning they should have given? Namely, that the amount of yeast MUST NOT be increased in the same proportion to any increase in volume, as customary with all unleavened mixtures. One MUST NOT use more. One MUST USE LESS. Not three or five times more for three or five times more flour, but less. In short, although a rough rule is that 1 oz of yeast will leaven 3-4 lbs of flour, one does not increase the quantity in proportion to the flour used. An important deterrent to doing so is the fact that bread made with more than the necessary quantity of yeast will be poor in flavour, and become dry and stale more easily.

The action of yeast is always a variable. It is dependent on four combined factors- time, moisture, warmth, and the techniques used for dough making. It may be that, given time and the right conditions for growth of the yeast, half, or even a quarter, of that amount will do the work just as effectively. For yeast not only reproduces itself under such conditions, it stimulates a natural fermentation and maturing of the flour with which it is combined. Amounts recommended in books are only true for doughs of a very short rising period. The fact that there can be a great difference is amply demonstrated by the difference between the old professional bakers' use of 6 oz of yeast to a sack of flour for a long-time dough, compared to the modern bakers' 6 lbs of yeast per sack (16 times as much), for a no-time dough, or its equivalent in bread improvers.

Here are some simple rules.
1. The longer the time of leavening , the less the yeast.
2. Half, or even a quarter, the amount for long doughs as for short doughs.
3. Half for dried yeast as compressed. (Initial rising is fast.)
4. Even less for granular dried yeast, than for powdered dried yeast.
5. Caution should err on the side of less with amounts given on packets.
6. Less yeast in warm weather than in cold.
7. Do not heat above 54 degrees. Yeast cells will die.
8. Allow 15 minutes to come back to life in tepid water.
9. Do not use before it is fully dissolved.
10. Compressed yeast can be stored in refrigerator, covered with cold water.
11. Store packets of dried yeast in a cool dry place, e.g. the cold part of the refrigerator.
12. If dried yeast reacts badly, allow that it may be stale.

The French, for example, allow 1/3 oz. yeast for 2 lb of plain bread dough, or 1 lb of enriched type dough. If leavening goes wrong, a fresh boost of yeast can be added.

Another word of warning. If you do go back to old recipe books for hints, remember that home-made or bakehouse yeasts of long ago were not the same as commercial yeasts available today. The recipe that was right then may be wrong now. Yeasts now are much stronger, and recipes must be modified to allow for the difference. So, amateur baker, beware. If you are a simple novice, stepping into your kitchen for the first time, remember the force you are unleashing: the capacity of this most simple form of life, the single living cell, to create for us one of the great miracles of human life, the leavening of bread. Although too small to see, it is made up of a quantity of complex chemical substances.

What exactly happens in this process of fermentation called leavening, which makes bread so utterly different from the unleavened batters, cakes and biscuits? Yeast can be brought to life , even if dried, by adding it to tepid water, when it begins to reproduce itself. Well-fed yeast cells will reproduce a generation every five hours. The foods that suit yeast contain the elements of natural ferment in themselves, such as warm mashed potatoes, moistened flour and natural sugar. Therefore the yeast-laden liquid serves to stimulate the natural fermentation of the flour itself, when added to it. The yeast's action is twofold, both on the starch and the gluten protein of the wheat flour. Fermentation of the starch produces carbonic acid gas. This gas does not escape. In its efforts to do so, it spreads through the mass of the dough contained within the gluten, which expands as the gas does, trapping it in a myriad of tiny balloons, making the dough light, porous and spongey.

This capacity is obviously greater where the fraction of the gluten in the flour is higher rather than lower. It is higher in what are known as strong flours, with a gluten range of 12-15%, than in soft flours with a gluten range of 8-10%. Therefore, strong flours are usually used for bread-making, and soft flours for cake-making. The novice should beware of this need to distinguish in the choice of flours. She is just as likely to attempt to make bread with ordinary household flour intended for cakes, and wonder why she has a crashing failure. She should rather go to the bread shop in her friendly shopping centre (now around because of the development of the spiral oven), and ask for some bakers' flour in a smaller quantity than the fifty pound bags that I was obliged to buy.

Now, what flour will she need for a long-time dough? Does she automatically use strong flour? This is where the plot thickens. Were strong flours used by the British in the old days of their overnight baking? Or the French for their marvellous light, white breads? Or the Viennese for their famous Vienna bread? The answer is no. English and continental flours in those countries were usually soft, but even these differed, French soft flours being sweeter and stronger than the British. Only in more recent times has hard wheat been imported from Canada and America to blend with the softer Continental wheats to meet the demands of modern no-time dough bread-making with high mechanical beaters. Soft flour does not take kindly to short-time dough maturing, and rapid mechanical kneading or moulding. The home-baker can adopt a modified version of this by adding extra gluten from a health food shop to her soft flour bread mix.

Now you know the chancey factors involved- the kind of flour, and the kind of yeast- do not pause on the brink and turn back, but go to phase two. Ask what else is variable in the quantity or quality besides yeast.

1. LIQUID
(a) Strong flour absorbs more water than soft.
(b) New flour absorbs more water than old flour.
(c) Soft water makes a more lively bread dough easier to handle, but not necessarily a better bread.
(d) Rainwater makes the best bread of all. There are also rules for quantity.
(a) Two parts of flour to one of water makes good bread.
(b) 1 part of milk to 3 parts of water prolongs the life of a loaf.
(c) Half or all milk makes a better crust in all breads.
(Note - lard, butter, or cream will produce the same effect.)

Ultimately the ratio of liquid to flour depends on the particular flour, and the quantity of liquid that any given flour will absorb will depend on trial and error.

2. SUGAR
(a) No sugar for modern compressed yeast. It does not need it. Too long a direct contact between yeast and sugar can destroy yeast cells.

(b) A pinch of sugar as a starter for dried yeast.

(c) Ginger can be used instead of sugar.

Sugar can be used for sweet leavened pastries, buns, breads etc., but such recipes are irrelevant to this summary, as they are mainly short-time doughs. True brown sugar can distort flavour as well as colour.

3. SALT

Salt is not added merely for taste. It acts on yeast and dough during rising, and helps to retain moisture in the loaf.

(a) Do not decrease the amount during leavening, as for yeast. 1/2 oz per lb of flour; 5 oz to 11 lbs.

(b) Rock or sea salt is better than free running salt (with added magnesium carbonate.) Such salt should be dissolved in water.

A high proportion of salt acts on yeast and dough during rising and slows down its action, preventing it from over-fermenting and developing a sour taste. Less than one teaspoon of salt per pound of flour produces virtually unsalted bread.

4. FATS

(a) *BUTTER*

It should be not be worked in until after the first rising, as the fat globules will coat the particles of flour, impeding the action of the yeast. Butter is the best fat for bread dough, except for special white breads that may use thick, clotted cream. It gives bread a good crust and crumb.

(b) *CREAM*

Cream is often more satisfactory than butter for enriched yeast doughs, pastries and batters, giving a lighter, smoother texture, and being quicker and easier to work with; particularly thick, mature cream, even clotted cream, as in West Country recipes like Sally Lunns.

(c) *OLIVE OIL.*

This makes doughs extremely easy to knead for rolls, pizzas, etc. Other oils can subsitute.

(d) LARD.

This was commonly used for English muffin dough.

5 EGGS

(a) Eggs can have a drying effect, so use with caution.

(b) Treat eggs like yeast. Do not multiply them in ratio to volume of flour. This is the reason the older recipes prescribed volume not number.

6. FRUIT AND FLAVOURS
(a) Warm fruit before working into dough to obviate a deadening effect, and to ensure even distribution.
(b) Rub them with flour first to prevent sinking to the bottom.
(c) Mix fruit into the dough either initially, or after the first rising.
(d) Work in by hand, or with a broad wooden spoon.
(e) Ground almonds add moisture, flavour and texture.
(f) Currants and raisins are to be preferred to sultanas.
(g) Cut up peel as small as possible.
(h) Ginger was an old favourite in bread, both as a yeast stimulant, and for its flavour.

BENEFICIAL CONDITIONS FOR MAKING GOOD BREAD
1. TEMPERATURE
Moderate warmth is basic to the entire process of bread-making until it enters the oven. Remember that hot water has an adverse effect both on yeast and flour, and that dough will to a certain extent generate warmth itself.
(a) Water should be neither too hot nor too cold - 88-100 Fh or 37-43 C. It should be a little warmer in cold weather than in hot.
(b) Flour should be warmed, but not in hot weather.
(c) The bowl for mixing or the tin for baking a dough should be warm.
(d) The bowl for leavening should be well covered to obviate any draught.
(e) A very long-time dough (18 hours) can be left wrapped in cold water. (This method is also useful for raising dough in very hot weather.)
(f) If ice is added, it produces the holey texture of French bread, and a wafer-like crust. The dough may be put in a warm steamy bathroom.
(g) If left overnight, it may be brushed with oil to obviate a skin.
There are only two moments in the life of bread when it can tolerate extremes of temperature- that is when it is put into the hot oven to bake, and when it is stored in the freezer after it is cooled.

2. LEAVENING (OR PROVING) UTENSIL

The answers to this question of choice are unexpected.
(a) Cloth lined baskets upside down (a preferred French method).
(b) Shallow earthenware crocks, widening at the top.
(c) Terracotta pots (as for flowers.)
(d) A container for cold water leavening (dough in cheesecloth.)
        In the old days, bread dough was covered with warm sacks, and left to rise in wooden troughs with lids. Now it may be left to rise covered with a sheet of polythene held in place by a warm dish or plate. But this does not mean that dough can therefore be consigned to a polythene bag. This would not allow it to breathe.

3. BAKING UTENSILS

(a) Bakers' steel, or aluminium tin. Aluminium is a good heat
      conductor.
(b) A pyrex glass bowl.
(c) A terracotta pot, 5 1/2 inches by 4 1/2 inches (soaked in water
      overnight). The bread dough may be put inside it, or the pot may
      be turned upside down over it to make an oven within an oven.
      This makes an excellent crust, and a very evenly baked moist
      crumb.
(d) An earthenware pot either unglazed, or glazed inside but not
      outside—tempered by heating, oiled, in the oven twice—gives a
      more flavoursome loaf. (Not the type turned out by art potters!)
(e) A simple terracotta tile as a basis for a free-shape loaf with, or
      without, a cake hoop.
(f) A two handled casserole dish of the stock pot type
(g) An iron pot, such as the Irish use for their fruit breads.
(h) Austrian or German kugelhopf tins.
        The light metal tins for ordinary domestic baking are less satisfactory. Bread baked in, or on, such tins have a tough crust that is not acceptable. New red house tiles are better as a base. Indeed, such baking tins were unknown until the turn of the eighteenth century; such a system being rejected everywhere but in Holland and England.
        Loaves may generate a certain amount of steam in cooking. This effect can be enhanced by slashing the crests with a razor just before baking, and spraying water into the cuts. A bowl of water in the oven is unnecessary.

4. HOW TO MIX THE DOUGH

Elisabeth David, in her monumental book on bread, says, 'Some of the methods used by our ancestors, archaic though they may sound, still turn out more satisfactory than the newer fangles of our own age' (English Bread and Yeast Cookers p. 321.1.)

(a) Have all measuring equipment ready. Scales, jugs, thermometers.

(b) Warm water to tepid heat.

(c) Put yeast in warm water to cover. Add a pinch of sugar, if dried, unless the yeast is 2 ozs or more.

(d) Stir and leave 10-15 minutes until a frothy cream has developed.

(e) Warm flour and mixing bowl while yeast is dissolving in warm water. Combine one part of water to 2 parts of flour.

(f) Whisk for a few seconds, then mix into the dough.

(g) Mix the dough with hands, sprinkling with more flour if too sticky and wet to work.

(h) Work the dough until it is lithe and elastic, and comes away easily from the sides of the bowl. Form into a ball, and sprinkle with flour.

(i) Cover with polythene, and a warm dish or plate. Leave to rise.

(j) Leave overnight, or all day. At the end of that time, knock it down with a good punch. Gather it up and slap it down on the board hard several times. Knead on a floured board by pushing it out, and folding it over itself in a three-cornered fashion. Repeat 3-4 minutes, or longer for quantity.

(k) Put into a baking utensil to rise again. This second proving will be quicker, and the volume greater.

(l) When risen to the top of the tin, or within 1 1/2 inches in the case of a terracotta pot, put into oven.

As a footnote to this list of steps in making a dough, it should be added for the benefit of the newcomer to this dough-making ritual that the importance of punching down and knocking back a dough lies in the fact that it creates a redistribution of the gas bubbles, and reinvigorates the yeast to form new air balloons. Furthermore, it is important to note that butter should not be worked into the dough until after the first rising, or the fat globules will coat the flour particles making them sticky, and impeding the action of the yeast. This is not a problem when the yeast has been allowed time to act. Olive oil is especially good for rolls and small

154

bread, as it makes the bread very easy to knead. Lard is good for muffin dough and pizzas.

5. THE OVEN

Modern domestic ovens have never been as adequate as the special brick and tile special baking ovens in every farmhouse. They gave a very uniform heat, which domestic ovens seldom do with several degrees difference in heat between the top and the bottom. Correct heat is supremely important. Bread should never be baked below an initial heat of 400, or a minimum of 205. A fan-forced oven with even heat all round is ideal.

(a) Loaves generally take an hour to bake.
(b) The baking heat should be by two stages. The first stage should be 30 minutes at 425-450 (220-230) degrees. The second stage should be 15 minutes at 400 (205) degrees. The third stage may be 15 minutes reducing to 350 (180) degrees. (The bread may be slipped out of its container, and turned on its side at any time after the first stage).
(c) Changing the position of the bread in the oven may be advantageous, unless the oven is fan-forced.
(d) If the bread has not been removed from the tin for the last stage of baking, remove immediately at the end of baking. Do not leave in tins otherwise it will become sodden.
(e) Keep in earthenware crock, or freezer, but not in the refrigerator.

155

6. STORAGE

(a) Do not store until cool. Then in a dry mould-free container.
(b) Allow to breathe if it is in a earthenware crock. Airhole in cover, or lid raised with a cork.
(c) If storing in a freezer, compress air from freezer bag, and close well.
(d) If possible, do not store in a refrigerator. It draws the moisture.
(e) For the short term, wrap in a clean dry cloth, or invert bowl over a platter.

7. BREADS MADE IN COMBINATION WITH OTHER INGREDIENTS

(a) *POTATO BREAD.*
Equal quantities of warm mashed potatoes and wheaten flour. Excellent in flavour and lightness.
Best for toast. Rising takes longer than usual. Baking is at a lower temperature. More salt is needed than for ordinary bread. (Potatoes are rubbed into the flour as with fat.) Victorian bakers often used a small proportion of potato mash in doughs as a fermenting agent, and not, as was alleged, to adulterate the flour. Potato is second only to rice in keeping bread moist.
(b) *PUMPKIN BREAD.*
As above. In both cases, compress excess water out of the vegetable.
(c) *RICE BREAD.*
2 lbs of warm, cooked rice to 28 lbs of flour=10 loaves. Excellent moist, light honeycombed texture.
Best for sandwiches. Mix the dough in the usual way. Add a little more flour, if too soft, when knocking down. If baking is too hard, with too much colour, cover with an inverted casserole. The Greeks make an 'orinde' rice bread . Rice flour is best for dusting any dough at the moulding stage.
(d) *SOYBREAD.*
A proportion may be used to enrich white flours nutritionally.

8. OTHER TRADITIONAL BRITISH FOODS

1. Oats were staple meals in Scotland, English Midlands, and border counties, so flat griddle-baked oatcakes, such as bannocks, or haver cakes, as they were known, were common. These, like the muffins, were often yeast-leavened. They were usually thin, cooked very slowly, and took a long time in preparation.
2. Barley Bannocks were made in the same way as oatcakes, and were far more common than oven baked loaves. Even where there were old primitive clay ovens, as in Devon, Cornwall and parts of Wales, barley loaves continued popular, as barley was said to give a better colour and keeping qualities in the loaf. Sopen barley bread could be very dark. Barley meal pancakes, leavened with yeast, were said to be most delicious.
3. Buck-wheat pancakes, like Russian Blinis, were well known in the Midlands. These are made with 6 oz flour, 1 oz yeast, 8 eggs and milk.

9. TWO MODERN FASHIONS

1. BRAN

For centuries, the bran of wheat was not considered wholesome. It was fed to horses and pigs, except in times of famine, when 'bran tea', made from boiling the bran was mixed with the dough, and the rest was still fed to the animals. People, whether high or low, believed only white bread was fit for human consumption. They would have agreed with the words of the 'Dyetary of Health' 1542, which said 'bread having too much bran is not laudable'. When people once spoke of good bread, they were not only speaking of its digestive qualities, but success in baking. Good bread, in that sense, could not be readily made from flour, when the bran layers of the outer skins of the grain were still adhering to the endosperm flour. These layers could discolour the flour and spoil its baking qualities. Doctors did not begin to press for inclusion of wheat bran in household bread on health grounds until the middle of the nineteenth century, and met with strong opposition from the flour mills. The millers disputed the need to eat wholemeal bread in order to have a satisfactory fraction of fibre in the diet. But the doctors replied that fibre from other

157

sources was not as satisfactory as cereal fibre, an assertion just as debatable today as it was then.

2. MALT

Malt sprang into favour late in the nineteenth century for various reasons.

(a) As a bread improver. By this was meant an effect on the moisture, volume, crust and bloom of a loaf.
(b) As a medicine to ward off colds, flu and other ills.
(c) As a replacement for flavour lost by the exclusion of germ and bran from modern roller-milled flours.

The craze was so great that almost everything that could be malted was malted; such as cocoa, marmalade, and jellies. I can certainly remember being obliged to eat a dark sticky substance called 'Robelene' off a spoon. The craze is, of course, still with us.

In conclusion of this segment on long-time doughs, let me give that great cookery writer, Elisabeth David, the last word, 'In old days bread doughs were given much longer and slower fermentation than today's high speed doughs. The true essence of good bread lies in the slow ferment and unhurried ripening of the dough' (Op. cit pp. 97/100).

POSTSCRIPT

Even as I put this manuscript aside without baking the two loaves Dr. Zentner suggested, Professor Fraser rang to tell me he had found the article to which Dr. Zentner referred in the September 23 issue of the 'New Scientist' and was sending it to me. In his covering letter, he remarked 'this one I think refers to your family's problems'.

I read the theory of Furth & Harding with dumbfounded approval certain of its advice exactly tallied with my own over many years, and its warning - stated in the headline summary - 'When you drink a large glass of juice, or eat a chocolate bar on a empty stomach, your blood stream becomes awash with sugar. The longer this lasts the worst it is for your proteins. Evidence is growing that sugars cause serious damage to long-lived proteins.'

Long-lived proteins? What on earth are they you will say as I did? Glycation end products the article informed me, known whimsically by doctors as AGES, because they are thought to accumulate in the aged. Three important types of long-lived proteins are crystallins in the lens of the eye, myelin in the nerve sheath, and collagen in skin, tendon and basement membrane (of capillaries etc.) There is also haemoglobin, the protein that carries oxygen in the blood.

Glycation, it seems, was first identified by Louis Maillard in 1912 in relation to the bread industry. He worked out the three stages by which proteins turn brown when sugars attack them, and therefore how to minimise this reaction which adversely affected bread's flavour, appearance and volume.

How then does glycation affect the quality of life in humans? Because it causes proteins to malfunction by upsetting 'the balance of charge groups on the protein's surface, altering the way it interacts with water and other molecules.'

The consequences mentioned are quite alarming, namely -
1 Impairment of fat and cholestoral physiology leading to coronary heart disease.
2. Depressed ability of immunoglobulin G (the most common anti-body) to deal with the bacterial toxins.
3. Loss of capacity of blood albumin to bind to long-chain fatty acids.
4. Impaired ability of collagen to form lining structures of

capillaries.

The prime condition for glycation is said by these authors to be a high level of glucose over several hours - most likely to occur in diabetics; more likely to occur in the ageing; and capable of occurring in all ages if sugars are taken on a empty stomach in any form - juices, sweets, chocolates.

Damage is slow, and can occur over many years leading to such conditions as the cataracts or circulatory disease of diabetics, skin damage and heart disease of the aged. In this context the authors are emphatic, 'The damage of cataracts can be quite specifically linked to sugars'. A human lens will go cloudy in a concentrated solution of glucose like a lens afflicted with a cataract.

The authors stress the fact that glycation is not avoided simply by eliminating sugar (sucrose) from the diet, as most health purists insist on doing. If anything it compounds the problem, as I have so often said, in that glucose is substituted for sugar. They point out that a can of Lucozade (a British sugar free drink) contains 65 grams of free glucose, which is higher than the amount given for a glucose tolerance test and there is nearly as much glucose in half a litre of unsweetened fruit juice as in a Mars bar. They also mention that fructose is a very dubious substitute for reasons not yet fully researched.

I read their final conclusion with weary content. It had been such a long and patient wait to read those words written by someone other by myself, words I had first set down over twenty years earlier that we are all well advised "to take carbohydrate as part of a mixed meal with protein, fat and fibre, and to avoid high-sugar snacks on an empty stomach".

And yet even now a question may be on their answer. I had argued that fermented and well processed starches were more digestible and less damaging both in children and adults. But in terms of the glycation argument, such starches would be more readily converted to glucose than their original carbohydrate with the symptoms described, raising glucose levels in the blood, but this did not seem to be the case. Therefore, I could only support a qualified interpretation of their argument in the 'New Scientist', and refer to the differential effect on glucose levels depending on which starch was involved. This is reflected in the comparative graph at the beginning of this book, ranging from glucose and maltose as the most troublesome sugars down to fructoseas the least.

I had long wondered if the long processing of proteins, I advocated as part of the folk wisdom of food, modified the proteins in some significant way, and if so whether this could decrease the risk of glycation. But of course I have no answer for such a question. So again despite the blinding light of this article, a darkness of ignorance still lies beyond.

While I wait for researchers to move forward down that laborious road they follow, I will at once start taking aspirin, which is considered to prevent the first step in the glycation process plus the vitamin C and E recommended by Wolff, who has an alternative theory that glucose combines with oxygen producing auto-oxidation. But what awful outcome flows from this the article does not say.

A bet each way? Why not? Hope springs enternal. So with my last bow, dear reader, I say good luck wherever your betting lies. In my case, it will lie with the theory of Furth & Harding, which so much better fits my facts. I will go my way with the new buzz word 'glycation' on my lips, as it no doubt will soon be on yours.